TOTAL BODY FITNESS

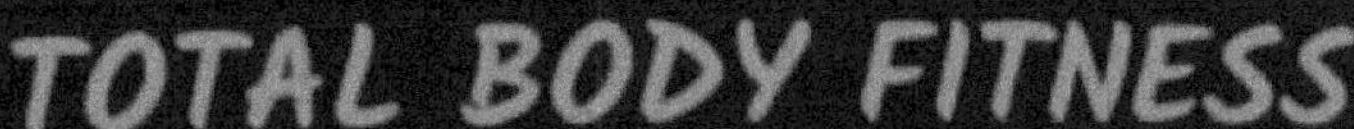

WAY TO GO FOR YOUR BODY FITNESS WITHOUT STRESS

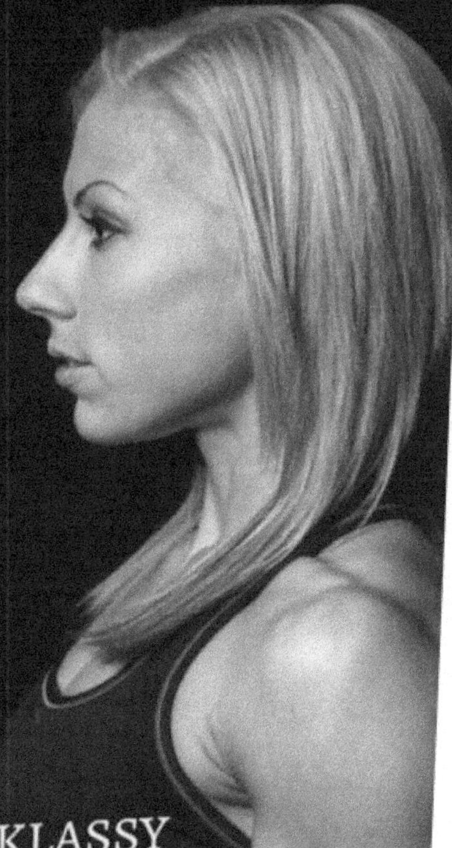

ALL KLASSY

TABLE OF CONTENT

BUYER BEWARE: DON'T BUY THESE ELLIPTICAL TRAINERS

WATER AND EXERCISE

HOW CAN I FIND THE BEST ELLIPTICAL TRAINER?

Fitness And Where You Stand Right Now

The ability to maintain the finest possible physical shape is referred to as fitness. Then, you might wonder, "What am I exercising for?" This will mean different things to different people.

Most people's main concern is maintaining their health for as long as possible. Your body, you see, is built to function like a machine. The complete machine functions as effectively as it can when every component is taken care of. The machine won't run well and eventually won't run at all if it is partially or completely neglected.

For instance, an automobile will survive a lot longer if it is carefully maintained over a lengthy period of time. If it isn't maintained, like when the oil isn't changed, the lifespan of the vehicle is shortened by many years. That may seem expensive to you, but if you think of this as your body, neglecting your machine could be costing you days, weeks, or even years of your life (your body.)

Being fit is essential to living. Remember that fitness is something you can get into the habit of doing, which makes it easy, before we get on our soapbox.

You don't have to strain to be physically fit. You were probably instructed to wash your teeth when you were three. You acquired the ability to dress yourself. You probably despised it when you were learning how to perform them. However, after you mastered the technique, you no longer gave it a second thought. Do you stress out today about brushing your teeth? Not at all, it's just a habit. We want you to picture it when you think of fitness.

Simply said, it's something you do. It's true that getting fit and maintaining a healthy lifestyle will be the hardest in the beginning. You will fear it. You'll come up with reasons not to. You'll say that getting in shape is impossible. You simply cannot give up what you love. That is untrue.

In fact, you'll see that fitness is something you can easily master if you have the willpower to sacrifice for a few weeks in order to save your life.

Right now, look at yourself. Do you see anything? If you are self-conscious about any portion of your body, the likelihood is high that you are bothered by that part of your body because it is unhealthy.

Fitness is about more than just losing weight, despite the fact that this is why many individuals first become interested in it. Knowing where you stand on these variables will help you take steps to enhance your general health, lengthen your life, and improve the quality of the life you are now leading.

It's wonderful if you don't believe you need to lose weight. You have made progress toward good health. But that doesn't mean you don't have health issues that go beyond that. Although they aren't officially overweight, many people are still at risk for high blood pressure, high cholesterol, and other issues. You must therefore take into account the fact that improving general health is crucial.

What's Healthy?

Your weight, blood pressure, and body mass index are accurate measures of your general health.

But it goes far beyond than that. You need to be conscious of how your body is operating. Do you have any physical limitations? This could be a topic to consider if you physically find it difficult to lift anything out of worry about hurting your back.

If you experience any problems with your arms, legs, neck, or other body parts, you should address these specific problems. The best place to start is to discuss with your doctor the causes of your lack of physical fitness in those areas. You can improve your overall health by doing this, and as a result of learning how, you can also improve your situation.

Your diet has a significant impact on your health. Your body gets the energy it needs from food to complete the tasks you give it. When viewed through the lens of a machine, food provides your body with the fuel it needs to function.

If you don't give it wholesome meals to eat, it won't perform effectively. Have you ever filled up your automobile at a gas station only to discover that the fuel wasn't satisfactory or even good quality? Your car lags as a result of that. Because you don't get the gas mileage you are used to, you could even need to do more maintenance on your car than usual.

Eating well is equally important for how your body works. If you regularly eat the worst foods, your body won't perform as well as it would if you constantly ate the best foods.

Without nourishment, your body could become ill more quickly and severely. Your body doesn't heal from wounds as quickly.
Your blood pressure increases, and your heart rate increases to risky levels. You are more susceptible to limitations of the body and mind.

Numerous problems result from eating an improper diet of foods. But what is health exactly, and why is it important?

Produce is one of the foods with the greatest nutrients. Due to their exceptionally low calorie count, they provide significant antioxidant quantities that aid in your body's healing process, improve your general level of physical fitness, and enable you to consume more.

Fruits, which are sweet, can fulfill a sweet craving. They also provide you with a variety of minerals and antioxidants that provide your body with the energy it needs.

Products made from whole grains should be a part of any wholesome diet. Compared to "white" foods, whole grains are far healthier for you. In contrast to other things, they don't cause you to gain weight. You may still enjoy your favorite flavors without adding extra calories, fats, or sweets that could be harmful to your health by making minor adjustments to everyday items like bread, spaghetti, and potatoes.

Consuming water is also essential. People who don't drink enough water find that instead of losing water, their bodies retain it. Your body starts to become dehydrated, which compels you to drink as much liquid as you can. Your body will be properly hydrated, you'll eat less, and other liquids won't have as many calories if you drink enough water.

Significant amounts of meat are also a part of the diet. To get the protein you require, you should abstain from eating fatty meats. By switching to a diet that exclusively consists of lean foods, you can lower your intake of cholesterol, which will eventually clog your heart and restrict blood flow to the rest of your body.

You just need to improve in these five areas, that's all. The good news is that it usually doesn't take much work to make things happen.

How Can You Improve?

Your body can only function and move better if you make it better. Although first difficult, it will become simpler. Exercise is a key component of our total fitness improvement strategy, along with the other fitness components discussed later in this book.

Although many individuals detest exercise, keep in mind that your body was not designed to sit in a chair at a computer all day. According to estimates, the majority of individuals don't get the recommended amount of exercise, which can result in a variety of health issues.

Again, chances are likely that you aren't getting enough exercise and fitness into your life even if you aren't overweight. To increase your health and fitness, you must use and build your muscles.

Okay, it's time now. Right after that comes the horrible, restrictive diet that will forever dull your taste senses.

NO! The majority of food that is accessible that is in its natural state is perfectly healthy for you, so you don't have to be constrained by what you can eat! If you give it a shot, you could even discover that you prefer these foods to the high-fat, high-cholesterol ones you're currently eating.

Foods play a major role in why individuals are unhealthy, thus changing your diet is essential to getting healthier. If you are unwilling to make adjustments in this area, your diet and fitness could endanger your health and cause you to die young.

But over time, a balanced diet can help undo a lot of the harm caused by eating the wrong things. That's exactly what you should aim for in this situation.

How can you increase the health of your mind? There are lots of fantastic ways to accomplish this. Recall how we claimed this exercise program would be enjoyable? Here are lots of fantastic, enjoyable ways to strengthen your emotional and mental health.

Every element is distinct in and of itself, as well as in the ways that it will enhance your overall well-being and physical fitness. You'll notice differences in how you feel and how you perceive the world if you incorporate as many of these things into your life as you can.

You must provide your body with the necessary physical movement in order to increase its physical fitness. This entails giving it the appropriate movement schedule.

Start by incorporating exercise into your day by doing strength and aerobic training. Visit the community or recreation center in your neighborhood. These activities can even be started at home, which will facilitate and enhance your enjoyment of the process.

Consider these quick and enjoyable ways to get the exercise you require to make it even better.

Put a pattern to it. If you try to accomplish it alone, your chances of success increase by 80%! Find a coworker to assist you!

Take your partner for a brief stroll outside after dinner. Take the kids along if you are unable to leave them behind. This is a fantastic way to spend time with loved ones without watching television.

If you are unable to get away from the TV, try a stationary bike. Riding the bike while watching your preferred TV. Time will fly quickly as you obtain the necessary exercise while still watching television.

Play sports and engage in other physical activities you like. Exercise can be gotten in by swimming, playing with the kids, or even joining a sports team without feeling like it.

Exercise and movement are necessary for full physical fitness. When you start incorporating them into your day, you'll probably come up with all kinds of reasons not to. However, you will start to like working out. It may be a lot of fun and a terrific way to relieve tension for many people. Make it a point to design an exercise that you will genuinely love. It will have a major impact on how successful it is for you.

Here are the pointers you need to launch your diet and exercise program and significantly enhance your health!

Boost your fruit and vegetable intake. Look for veggie recipes on your favorite recipe websites that don't rely heavily on sauces, butter, or creams. Each week, include one new recipe in your diet.

Start seeking leaner beef cuts. Keep in mind that saturated-fat-rich meats block your heart. A tasty substitution is ground beef. Instead of using beef, try using ground turkey or pork in place of at least some of the beef. The difference in flavor won't be discernible. Eat more pork, chicken, and fish instead of beef.

portions should be smaller. A single serving of food shouldn't be bigger than your hand in size. Eat a little more slowly to prevent feelings of hunger.

To find recipes that are good for your heart, go to the American Heart Association website. Try to find ways to make your present recipes better by substituting healthier ingredients for butter, salt, and unhealthy meals. Examine your grains. Use whole grain pasta and rice instead of white. Switch to full grain bread from white bread.

Take Coke out of your diet. Your health will significantly improve only from this one simple activity. Your body gains weight, and it poses a variety of long-term health problems.

Check the labels. To find out what is in the things you eat, learn to read the labels. Eat fewer foods that are high in fat, cholesterol, and sugar.

You should think about cutting calories if you need to reduce weight. You need to eat less and exercise more if you want to lose even a tiny amount of weight. Simply eating less and exercising more each day is a trendy diet that is safer and more effective overall.

You can't choose not to eat healthfully if you want to live

longer and be healthier. Even if you enjoy cooking, you shouldn't put off learning to make healthier recipes because you are too busy, don't like those foods (you probably have no idea what they taste like anyway!), or think it will take too much effort.

Live requires food, and maintaining a good diet is crucial to living a long life. For the sake of convenience, speed, or habit, don't compromise here. Although making adjustments can be difficult at first, it is guaranteed that once you get into the habit, you will love the changes you have made

Exercise Balls- Everything you want to know

What is this ball exactly?

With the help of these balls, you can perform a variety of exercises in novel ways. Exercise balls are incredibly stylish to capture your attention. The benefit of these balls, which were imported by a group of Swiss medical therapists, is that they may be used as an alternative kind of support when exercising.

The primary goal

Your body's major muscles become stronger and more toned as you exercise with these balls. They are great for various yoga positions, using weight training equipment, or using dumbbells for muscle toning because they feature textures that are obviously exceptionally soft.

Fundamental benefit

These training balls have the advantage of holding their shape under intense pressure and being equally durable. You can find information on the weight and load values that these balls can truly support in the manuals that come with them. Additionally, they give you soft yet solid support, which helps to completely rest your body.

Building Blocks of Exercise Balls

Exercise balls are available in a variety of colors and finishes. Alternatively, you might decide to get one based on the texture of your room. Depending on your inclination, you may easily store them under your bed or a table. They may be viewed as playthings by kids when not in use. Children playing with them won't suffer any harm because they are soft and non-toxic.

Medical benefit

They were primarily created to support the body while you exercised. This served as the inspiration for its design and was the original medicinal therapy. As you workout, you can keep your equilibrium. Regardless of how your body is positioned! These balls are made of burst-proof latex or another substance that is nonetheless safe to use.

Universal usefulness

Only with the use of these training balls is it possible to perform a number of yoga and muscle toning postures. These exercise balls are quite useful for this. Exercise balls include stability components that traditional floor exercises do not. When these balls are utilized, muscles that are passive during general exercise immediately become active and strengthen. For the treatment of any common backaches or spinal diseases, exercise balls are quite helpful. When the spine and these exercise balls are adjusted in harmony, back aches are typically lessened.

After a string of backaches, exercise balls would assist folks resume their regular activity. Additionally, increased muscle strength results in increased flexibility. The muscles thereon would function more effectively due to the movement in the spine caused by these balls.

The next time you intend to exercise really, be sure to give an exercise ball a try. When exercising with it versus not, you'd feel a difference in comfort.

Elliptical trainers from New Zealand have added intense competition among all currently available brands of elliptical trainers throughout the world, especially in the United States of America. These elliptical trainers are just as trustworthy as the most expensive and sophisticated elliptical trainers, but they are more reasonably priced and guarantee to offer comparable characteristics to their rivals. You shouldn't be surprised by what you discover as you examine them. This article will present two distinctive elliptical trainers made in New Zealand, comparing their features, quality, and pricing to those of competing companies in the market.

Nit-Trac 7-8200 Pro

This is the New Zealand-made elliptical trainer that is most frequently mentioned. Nit-Trac 7-8200 Pro would give you significantly more benefits at a reasonable price than any other machine of its like. They offer a variety of workouts that can help someone maintain their bone density, cardiovascular training, real elliptical motion with low impact, and an all-around workout for the lower and upper bodies. These are just a few of the benefits of elliptical cross trainers. With just these qualities, this trainer stands apart from the competition in every country, including the United States.

This elliptical trainer, which is made in New Zealand, includes a large LCD screen, large non-slip pedals, roughly sixteen magnetic resistance levels, well-built, consolidated parts, and many other features that meet user needs.

The unmatched weight capacity of this machine is 330 pounds, which is unquestionably extremely well. This feature is superior to many of its American counterparts since it is the best of its kind for elliptical trainers. When compared to comparable elliptical trainers that cost between a thousand and ten thousand dollars, these New Zealand-made trainers fall into the category of best bargains.

E-Bike Elliptical Cross

This is Another New Zealand-made elliptical trainer. Although it lacks the premium features that the majority of the other New Zealand elliptical trainers would provide, it is an excellent alternative.

absolute bargain at the price it is being offered. Eight resistance levels, a huge LCD display, and a couple sizable, slip-resistant pedals are all included. It also has built-in transport wheels, which facilitates the machine's easy movement, among other distinctive features. It also includes an adjustable handle bar post. This enhances the ease of the device. In addition, e-bike Elliptical Cross is a smart decision when compared to other Elliptical trainers in its price range because it costs less than $600.

After seeing them, you can be sure that the New Zealand Elliptical Trainers offer excellent value for your money because they also have unmatched features. These elliptical trainers from New Zealand have established themselves in the market due to their competitive pricing in the category. Try the New Zealand machines for your home as an alternative if you're looking for one.

All About Smooth Elliptical Trainers

The Smooth elliptical trainers are currently the most well-known brand and the best-selling elliptical trainer manufacturer on the Internet. These trainers were created by Smooth Fitness, which has been expanding their product line with new versions. You can learn more about Smooth in this article, including what makes them stand apart from other elliptical trainer brands. They are the most popular and well-liked products on the market.

The most obvious characteristic of Smooth elliptical trainers is the price they have assigned to the services they provide. These elliptical trainers don't belong in the budget-friendly or even the pricey category of purchases. In essence, they are considered mid-priced goods. Smooth running shoes don't cost more than $2,000 per pair. Precor's elliptical trainers are more expensive than Smooth's. However, when you contrast the two items, you will see that Smooth is significantly less expensive and that both elliptical trainers have comparable functionality. Because Smooth offers the most value for the money, it is for this reason that customers choose them over all other options. They compete with elliptical trainers, which cost over $3,000 yet offer comparable features.

Compare the Trainers

Additionally, Smooth's elliptical trainers include proprietary technology. Your height could be taken into account while adjusting the elliptical motion. You can burn more calories on an elliptical machine when your body is properly positioned. The majority of the time, incorrect motion alignment will prevent you from losing weight. By reducing the likelihood of injuries, proper alignment would also make these elliptical trainers safe to use. Because they offer improved functionality at a fair price, they are therefore chosen over other devices.

Other significant characteristics of these elliptical trainers include upper body arms that contribute to full body workouts, electromagnetic breaking, pulse sensors embedded into the hand grips, and larger weight capacities. Smooth Elliptical trainers are the most popular among people due to these and additional qualities. It is desirable since they also have noise controls. Numerous customer evaluations claim that the Smooth Elliptical Trainer is completely silent. The whisper mechanics of these trainers allow for a low noise system.

Similar to conventional brake systems, the electromagnetic brake system has fewer parts and no engine.

These elliptical trainers use current technology and have excellent warranties due to their wonderful features. Its improved user ratings are a direct result of this. Due to their excellent value for money, these elliptical trainers are frequently chosen by those with tighter budgets who cannot afford the most expensive models. You can get all the benefits of a high-end elliptical machine at a fair price with Smooth Elliptical Trainers.

So, if you're considering elliptical trainers, be sure to check out Smooth Elliptical trainers. Examine its characteristics and contrast them with those of more expensive products. You would understand that Smooth Elliptical trainers are unquestionably a good investment.

When buying gym equipment, most individuals these days choose for multifunctional or all-in-one systems. However, there are various all-in-one system kinds.

Check the structure

Nowadays, a lot of people prefer not to purchase gym memberships in favor of spending money on a home gym. Any empty space in your home—even the solely the basement—could be designated as your home gym. In addition to helping you save money by integrating several gear kinds into a single machine, such equipment are also much lighter than individual machines, making it easier to store them in smaller spaces.

Before you consider purchasing all-in-one exercise equipment for your workout, examine your actual goals. Think about your goals for regular exercise and how an all-in-one piece of equipment might essentially help you.

Know the types

There are many different kinds of multipurpose exercise equipment on the market, and the majority of them are advertised in periodicals, on television, and online. The equipment that is regularly advertised is typically connected with people who prefer to lift weights.

Bowflex System

Currently, Bowflex and Total Gym are the two most widely used brands of multipurpose workout equipment. Instead of the conventional weights used for only lifting, the Bowflex system uses resistive bows that bend. Bowflex has been created to accommodate a wide range of needs and price points. It is widely adaptable and exceedingly well-liked.

Even if you decide to keep it under the bed, a basic Bowflex system may be kept in small, confined spaces. The larger, more expensive Bowflex versions typically compete with the gear seen in commercial gyms. These guarantee high-quality exercises with high-quality gear.

Total Gym system

Chuck Norris, a superstar in martial arts, and Christie Brinkley, a supermodel, have both promoted the Total Gym System. This versatile system, which uses gravity and resistance rather than conventional weights, is just as effective and less expensive as Bowflex. With Total Gym, you could modify it to perform different exercises that targeted various parts of your body, which is advantageous.

Check the attributes

When making the decision to purchase an all-in-one system, make sure to consider things like the system's features, brand, pricing, and the real users of the device. If everyone in your family intends to utilize the system, you should choose one on which everyone can agree. Never choose a machine with a complicated operating system that not everyone can use.

Other brands

Other than Total Gym and Bowflex, there are a number of other multipurpose exercise equipment brands on the market, such as Weider and others. Make sure to check various models before settling on any machine, and then select the one that meets your budget and provides you with the best value for your money.

Show Your Body Curve And Achieve Fitness Through Belly Dancing

In western nations, belly dance is popular among both adults and children. It is the finest approach to maintain the curves in the case of grownups, improving them even more. There are numerous belly dancing lessons to accommodate every student. It starts at the beginning level and progresses through the intermediate and advanced levels. Anyone who wants to learn belly dancing must select the class that best suits their experience and skill.

In the beginning, women did belly dance to tone their hips. It all began in the Middle East with the primary goal of making childbirth easier. This custom soon evolved into art, entertainment, and physical activity. More than thirty moves could be displayed by skilled belly dancers. When you first start belly dancing, you should be aware that you do not have to learn every move by heart. Due to the isolated nature of the body parts involved in this dance, you would just need to be aware of the proper movements. While doing this, pay attention to the musical rhythm.

What role does belly dancing play in the curve?

The belly dancing movements are distinct. Even though your hips are raised, pushed, and shimmered, the tummy should roll and your pelvic muscles should be tilted. You would therefore be able to manipulate your arms like a snake. The legs either shimmy collectively or individually. Every movement needs to be practiced and mastered to produce a fantastic belly dance routine. After doing this, you can begin putting them into practice simultaneously or in many places. Soon after, there would be floor work where standing, sitting, and dropping would be taught. Additionally, a key aspect of belly dance is that many women prefer to play while wearing veils.

Skilled moves

Numerous aspects of it are highlighted by belly dance. Each of these motions has a different name according to different trainers, but they are all just expert movements. All of these physical movements—body quake, lock, thrust, shake, curve, and drop—must be related to belly dancing. Your hands, arms, and legs take control as fluid action is displayed. Real beautiful costumes are worn by belly dancers, allowing ladies to flaunt their curves. For manufacturing, more skin should be exposed.

sensual gestures by exposing her hips and midriff, the dancer demonstrates her craft and grace to the audience.

Belly dancing- form of exercise

In addition to being a form of art, belly dance is a beneficial form of physical activity. You strengthen your body's muscles while dancing, making it more fit.

In fact, including this dance in your everyday exercise routine is a terrific idea. Try some of the yoga stretches or use exercise balls when stretching. As a result, you should concentrate on fundamental hip, waist, shoulder, thigh, and belly movements.

Make sure you belly dance at least five times a week for 30 to 40 minutes to make it a beneficial exercise. If you incorporate belly dancing into your fitness routine in addition to a good diet and balanced lifestyle, you may be able to reduce or maintain your weight.

If you're one of the select few who wants to maintain fitness and have attractive curves, belly dance is the ideal activity for you to try.

The majority of asthmatics may doubt their ability to exercise correctly or safely. Despite what most people believe, even if you have asthma, you can still exercise to get in shape.

Chronic lung conditions like asthma are more often characterized by symptoms including coughing, wheezing, chest tightness, and shortness of breath. People who are genetically or environmentally susceptible to certain situations develop asthma.

Any attack could be started or made worse by triggers such viral respiratory illnesses, contact with cockroaches or dust mites, or exposure to allergens.

The following steps could be taken to prevent asthma:

1. Ensure that your pets are bathed at least once every week.

2. Never smoke or allow others to smoke inside your home.

3. When there are higher levels of pollen or mold, make sure to stay indoors with air conditioning.

4. Remember to wash bedding and stuffed animals in hot

water at least once a week.

5. Consistently wash your hands whenever you have the opportunity.

6. Get a flu vaccine for yourself.

7. In the winter, cover your lips and nose with a scarf.

8. Take initiative by becoming aware of your triggers and learning how to prevent them.

You are now aware of how to prevent asthma thanks to the aforementioned tips. There are also exercises that are appropriate in certain situations. Any doctor would advise continuing with sports and exercise,

whatsoever. All that is required of people is that they stay vigilant and wise about taking extra precautions to prevent attacks.

Doctors concur that taking an inhaler coupled with the necessary drugs is the best method to prevent attacks while you are exercising. When participating in an exercise session or a game, inhalers should not be used more than three times. It is advised to do easier exercises the next day if you coughed and wheezed the night before.

The symptoms of Exercise Induced Asthma, or IEA, are distinct from those of generic asthma. The attack happens roughly 6-7 minutes after the initial attack and is frequently worse in cold, dry conditions.

There are many activities you can participate in even if you have IEA. Walking, riding, downhill skiing, swimming, and team sports are some examples of these activities. There are several things you may do to make sure you get the necessary exercise.

Asthma is a completely physiological condition that requires a comparable type of medical care. It is not something that exists in the mind. The greatest person to help you with the disease is your doctor; you need to guard against asthma episodes.

Make sure you're wise by being proactive and taking the proper meds when you need to. Never let asthma ruin your life; live it up and get some exercise like everyone else.

Exercise And
Sleeping Better

The main component is the physical activity you engaged in during the day, which would identify and support you in getting a good night's sleep. A body that is active during the day will likely relax better and more quickly at night.

Exercise on a regular basis would provide better sleep quality with seamless transitions between phases and cycles. You'd find it simpler to manage life's stress and problems as long as you kept up your daily workouts.

There is a clear correlation between the total amount of exercise and how much is felt later, according to studies and other research.

The idea is to provide the body enough stimulus during the day so that the energy level declines at night, therefore physical activity during the day needs to be increased.

The body needs a certain amount of physical activity to function properly. Making sure not to exercise at least two or three hours before night is another important precaution.

Time

Early evening or late afternoon is the best time to workout.

Prior to your body preparing for relaxation and bedtime, make sure you utilize all of your physical energy that is now in use.

Amount and duration

Always continue to make an effort to exercise for at least 30 minutes three to four times per week. Be sure to do anything basic or even just brisk walking. Strenuous action, such as running, could also be included as an alternative.

The important objective is to raise heart rate by improving lung capacity. Regular exercise would enhance both your physical and mental well-being. Add regular exercise to your daily schedule.

There are many more workout activities besides walking and running that you might incorporate into your daily plan to enhance your level of physical activity. Try cardiovascular activity as one of

the greatest solutions if falling asleep feels more or the same as a struggle.

Your aim should be to increase the amount of oxygen that enters your bloodstream when you exercise. There are many different kinds of aerobic exercises available overall. Biking, running, utilizing a treadmill, skipping, or even dancing are a few of the activities.

There are a few non-aerobic workouts that you may find helpful to address the forgetfulness issue. We've included a few of them below.

Yoga

One exercise that has a stimulating effect on the nervous system, particularly the brain, is yoga. It makes use of yoga positions and breathing techniques to improve blood flow to the brain. Additionally, regular and restful sleep patterns might benefit from this. You might unwind and get rid of all your stress and anxiety by doing yoga regularly.

Tai Chi

The term "Tai Chi" describes a centuries-old method of breathing and moving that was created by Chinese monks. Tai Chi involves slow, precise movements that are perfect for people with joint problems or who are unable to engage in strenuous aerobic activity. Tai chi encourages relaxation to treat insomnia.

Small Crunches

If you don't feel like you have enough time to exercise every day, try to squeeze in a few minutes of exercise during your busy day. When possible, make sure to use the stairs instead than the elevator. Small things like these can do wonders for your body.

Make sure to park your car somewhere near the location so you may walk the extra block or two there. Numerous other minor things would be added to and expand the activity in your life. The main objective is to lead a balanced, healthy life that includes getting enough sleep.

Exercise And Your Complexion

Numerous benefits of exercise include improved complexion. Learn how the appropriate exercises may do wonders for your complexion.

Exercising knowledge

As is well known and reported, proper exercise can help you look and feel good. By exercising, you can maintain a healthy weight, increase your energy, and tone your muscles. The fact that exercising improves your complexion is something that many people are unaware of. Regular exercise could help you get the complexion you want.

Regular exercise will provide your skin with nutrition, oxygen, and new blood. Toxins are taken out of your body and important organs, especially the epidermis, are improved when there is abundant blood flow and optimal blood circulation, which directly result from performing the necessary workouts.

Sweating miracles

Many individuals believe that sweating causes breakouts of acne or pimples. Basically, sweating helps promote the flushing out of various pollutants from the epidermal layer, which cleans all the pores, and is helpful for any form of congested skin. Vigorous exercise may be able to eliminate the hormonal imbalances, trouble spots, and blemishes. Additionally, it would lessen the likelihood of an outbreak.

Acnes

Exercises that involve movement, such as jogging, biking, yoga, boxing, pilates, spinning, etc., can assist to lower chronic stress. This would actually stop the causes of acne brought on by stress.

Always remember that exercise is not a magic fix for all problems. Even while the acne would get less severe over time and linger for a shorter period of time, there would still be occasional outbreaks.

Aged skin

In certain cases, exercising is beneficial for skin disorders other than just acne. As we age, it is very typical for our skin to thin out, become less robust, or lose its elasticity, which are all indicators of aging. Skin tightening is aided by exercise.

Collagen is lost as we age, giving the face a very weary appearance. The majority of people are unaware that physical activity encourages healthy collagen growth within skin cells, plumping up facial skin and giving a younger, more vibrant appearance.

Unwind with Wrinkles.

Some people worry that wrinkles will irritate them. In these situations, folks should unwind after working out. Your muscles, particularly those in your face, will soften as a result of this. Then, on the other hand, would assert that your facial wrinkles would appear lightly emphasized, contributing to the young appearance you would always like.

With exercise, you can have a slim waist, more toned muscles, softer skin, fewer blemishes, and an overall younger, fresher appearance. You must be committed to your workouts if you want to alter or add to your complexion. Exercise would help you feel more alive and would also benefit your physical health. One would just need to make a small amount of time available in their schedule for exercise.

Working out for Extreme Fitness

One would need to exercise diligently for any type of extreme fitness because there are no justifications in these situations.

When people leave the gym, most of them ponder if giving up on life is comparable to bulking up. Such individuals spend a lot of time in the gym, just like a monk would in a monastery. They may have believed that the only way to shape your body into nothing less than a scorching, muscular physique is to spend hours each day, throughout the year, toiling away at the rusted iron.

It's certainly not necessary. Without a question, putting in a lot of effort is necessary to achieve exceptional fitness. Complete-body exercises could help someone advance because they are simple to fit into a regular plan. When you want to get extremely active but find it tough to keep to a single exercise regimen, this becomes more convenient.

Due to their dedication to their goals, athletes frequently experience maximum muscular contraction from big weights because it includes real full-body workouts. It provides enough room for full recovery so that one can develop and keep working hard to prevent burnout from overtraining.

The information provided here will give you a general notion of entire body work out if you are considering a foray into extreme fitness.

Time saver

Working out the entire body or all over might save a lot of time. When you start doing full-body exercises, you'll need to go to the gym less regularly; perhaps once or twice a week would be more than enough.

Quality of exercise stressed

Another benefit of total-body exercises is this. When a person is ready to work out their complete body, they may just need to invest a few short, intense workout sessions totaling less than an hour. In full-body workouts, the emphasis is frequently placed on the quality rather than the amount or duration. Even the time allotment per individual is not taken into account.

Cardiovascular boost

Exercises that target the entire body improve cardiovascular health. For the hour-long practice, two to four sets are allocated for each body area. Following a rigorous workout, every hour-long session gets the heart and other cardio vascular systems beating quickly.

One must adhere to a set of regulations when engaging in full-body exercises after becoming pumped up.

There is only one training session every two to three days. This is simple. The best part of this is that you have more time that you could use for aerobic workout sessions. People frequently rely on cardio exercises at the end of each workout, but these rarely prove to be very effective.

Heavy weightlifting is highly recommended. Despite the fact that many athletes believe in light weight training, it largely remains a fiction. People talk about saving energy for other body parts that will subsequently be used in the training. No matter the program, it should be understood that when training is not intense, a person will not make their best improvement.

One exercise is stressed for each muscle group. This is not only very simple to do but also very significant. Implementing simple yet effective workout approaches would imply avoiding the need for multiple exercises for each individual body area.

It is always advised to exercise for a very little period of time. Resistance training frequently has an impact on your body's natural hormones that are linked to muscular growth. prolonged exercise would

Intense exercise and improved catabolic control would raise testosterone levels. The best of both worlds might be yours with just 60 minutes of exercise.

You would surely achieve exceptional fitness with such a potent and practical workout routine.

In the current climate, maintaining good health and fitness is crucial. Any form of exercise—cardio, yoga, at home or at a gym—would help you reach the necessary level of fitness as long as you exercise safely.

Get advice on how to exercise properly

1. Stop and Go

Your lower body muscles would be strained if you ran a full sprint. If you intend to participate in a sport that requires a full sprint, keep this in mind. Stop-and-go workouts are the best to combat this flaw. For example, jog for about 5 to 10 meters while slowing down, then run another 30 meters with around 80% of your effort. This process can be repeated approximately five times.

2. Bended Knees

Three out of every four ACL injuries happen when athletes turn or land. The chance of injury is significantly reduced, according to the Journal of the American Academy of Orthopedic Surgeons, JAAOS, when your knees are bent as opposed to straight.

3. Take a break

A heatstroke cannot be treated like a minor headache. Keep yourself cool and well-hydrated to prevent this. According to IPSM's Dr. Dave Janda, make sure the combined temperature and humidity are less than 160.

4. Purchasing suitable equipment

Training injuries could result from improperly sized or fitted gear. On appropriate equipment, more money is well spent.

5. Executing it properly

Bad equipment is just as bad as bad technique. Get sound guidance from trainers and other experts; it will be very helpful for your training and workouts.

6. Heading west; in whatever direction

Warming up is necessary before training or playing in multiple directions. Any motion you would actually make, such as moving forward, backward, sideways, etc. This would properly prepare your body.

7. Record your own video.

Mirrors and cameras do not lie. People that are knowledgeable about your training should be shown the video to help with your exercise regimen.

8. Relax your shoulders

Even in situations where the rotator cuff is somewhat manipulated, your shoulder functions could be disabled. Stretching could be incorporated to safeguard the rotator cuffs.

9. Swim in the morning

Plan your swimming sessions for the morning. Less contamination would result from fewer swimmers in the pool.

10. Keep yourself safe

According to a UNC-Chapel Hill study, wearing bespoke mouthguards could cut the risk of suffering different injuries by as much as 82 percent. Spend some money on a personalized mouth guard, and it will last for many years, protecting your grin and teeth.

11. Make your muscle smooth

Gather data on ultrasound-assisted needle treatment. The needle in this therapy is guided by ultrasonography. Ultrasound would break up calcifications, repair scar tissue, and smooth the bone. Out of twenty patients, thirteen have improved. It would only take a few minutes for this session.

12. Shop your shoes in the evening

Evening shopping is almost always a smart move. The feet typically become swollen after a full day of work, which is comparable to a situation after 3 miles of running.

13. Running off-road

The ankles are trained to be steady when the surface is unstable.

14. Know your location

Whether skiing or bicycling, be sure to first be aware of the way. When one is comfortable with the route being taken, injuries can be avoided.

15. Work out hard

According to a study published in the Journal of Sports Sciences, worry would cause a 3 degree decrease in peripheral vision and a 120 millisecond delay in reaction time. The seasoned athlete relies on the skills they have learned and practiced when the going gets difficult. By enabling wider vision, it helps people stay calm under pressure and enables them to see and respond more quickly.

Woman Fitness: Building Strength

Women's fitness has always been popular. There are some similar purposes, though.

Women yearn for a beautiful body. This pattern has persisted regardless of whether it is in Hollywood or elsewhere. However, there are numerous effective exercise plans available for ladies who want to lose fat effectively.

One of the most popular and successful forms of exercise among women is strength training. In addition to fat loss, it helps with a number of additional advantages. This includes enhanced balance, injury prevention, recuperation and rehabilitation, heart disease prevention, delayed aging process, increased bone density with restoration, metabolic density, mass gain and lean muscle, improved sports performance, along with improved figure and appearance.

Before starting any strength training program, always with your doctor. You would be properly fit and have the necessary safety as a result. Actually, amid everything else, creating routines for your fitness program is the difficult. However, if you make sure to abide by the fitness recommendations made by your teacher, you will surely improve the likelihood that your fitness regimen will be successful.

1. *Constantly remember that you can never strengthen muscles in a single day. It is necessary to follow an allocation of at least 24 to 36 hours*. Exercise on consecutive days can result in muscle damage, exhaustion, and overtraining.

2. *It is impossible to lose weight instantly. For instance, you cannot lose extra tummy fat by doing 100 crunches continuously*. Such ease is not possible with belly fat. Your body should first be completely de-fatted by sufficient rest, a healthy diet, and exercise.

3. *The body cannot be toned in one sitting. A step-by-step process must be followed. Always focus on only one set of muscles*. Once you've finished, you can go on to the next objective. In addition to freely using weights, you might also think about employing machines.

4. *To guarantee excellent outcomes, strength training regimens need to be frequent and consistent.* Make it a point to remember that gaining the weight took many years, so losing it may also take some time. While strength training, you need to make some lifestyle changes. It is necessary to replace good behaviors with bad ones.

5. *Changes in strength training are necessary every four to six weeks. In essence, this would keep the body from being bored and make exercise incredibly fascinating.*

Changes in exercise routines and intensity levels are crucial. Continuous procedures can fail to deliver the anticipated outcomes. It is implied that you will develop from regular exercise.

6. Clear goals must be established in order for strength training programs to be designed appropriately. It could involve gaining muscle, increasing hypertrophy, maintaining weight, or even losing fat. Depending on the goal you were trying to achieve, different approaches would yield different optimal outcomes. When deciding between gaining muscle mass and losing body fat, there would be a significant difference. To design the ideal strength training program for fitness, keep the correct goals in mind.

7. All of the major muscles should be worked out in any regular regimen at least once to three times per week. Chest, shoulders, triceps, biceps, calves, quads, abs, glutes, and hamstrings would all fall under this category. If one of the muscle groups is neglected, there will be an imbalance.

Women who adhere to the recommended rules and train consistently in a consistent manner could develop a good, effective strength training program. Having a secure and healthy physique is always safe. Always be prepared to achieve that beautiful shape you have always desired.

Fitness: Definitely Not A Waste Of Time

It is usually recommended to stick to a committed workout routine so that your lifestyle improves and you don't run any risk.

Simply said, being fit means being healthy. People should dedicate themselves to a fitness routine for the rest of their lives.

The body is more like a temple, according to the Bible. It then becomes your responsibility to look after it. This could be seen as a justification for maintaining good mental and physical health, which is a great deed.

Whatever the situation, it requires a lot of work, even through acts. No matter how much work you put in, the results will be evident in the fruits it produces. Except for a select few, not everyone has the opportunity to live a healthy and happy life.

The importance of exercising to stay fit cannot be overstated. People can fight off a number of illnesses, including fatal ones like heart disease, by exercising.

It is disappointing to see how many more people today choose to disregard physical activity. This is the cause of the widespread diseases that plague people today. It is not surprising to see the healthcare industry thrive and attract a large customer base. Sometimes, this occurs despite the patients' wishes and desires.

Nowadays, high school students rarely engage in the health and fitness activities recommended by the General Surgeon and Council of President on Physical Fitness. This includes the 33% of Americans who live nationwide.

As youth transition into adulthood, they bring with them a disrespect for and a lack of interest in physical health. As a result of the low resistance, this would result in an increase in the number of illness sufferers.

Only 58 percent of Americans, according to a research by the National Institute on Aging, are believed to follow a lifetime fitness plan. Additionally, this health program is carried out in free time. About 26% of them consistently do the lifetime fitness act. It happens a lot, roughly three times every week.

The need of committing to a lifetime exercise plan is continually emphasized. People now, more than ever, essentially ignore it. Many people even ignore the reality that exercise actually adds value to one's life.

The obvious causes of death in our nation include cancer, chronic respiratory diseases, chronic heart disease, unintentional injuries from accidents, and stroke. The Centers for Disease Control report the five diseases mentioned above as major life-threatening hazards on an annual basis.

If you give the issue some thought, you will realize that all of the causes are easily avoidable. Again, only if the populace pays attention to workouts and exercise will this be achievable. The dedication to exercise for the rest of one's life would make a ton of sense. However, this does not include fatal accidents.

A lifetime fitness program would not only include an exercise regimen but also stringent dietary guidelines.

When one becomes committed to a lifetime physical fitness regimen, life will undoubtedly be lengthened. When in good physical and mental health, one can enjoy life to the fullest while picking up more daisies.

Finally, individual preferences vary. It is apparent that there will be less pains in the long run if you commit to a lifetime exercise regimen out of concern for your health.

Many people wish they had a fantastic figure to show off. There are plenty aspiring fitness models.

Men and women of today's generation both harbor dreams of

becoming fitness models at certain points in their lives. Many of them spent a significant amount of time and energy trying to break into the "fitness modeling scene."

What it is and what does it require?

Fitness modeling is all about having a lean, athletic figure that one can be proud of, as this will draw more attention from the public. It revolves around making one's body more attractive and in good form. The ultimate goal of this is obviously attention garnering. Finding everything is like becoming noticed. However, what matters is always the caliber and kind of the attention you receive. Being a fitness model would need not just having a stunning, lean figure but also being in good health. The total shaping of a person, including both the body and the will, is more important.

There are always many aspirants and hopefuls in the modeling industry. You must be tough enough to look straight at the facts if you truly wish to enter such a crowded field. For this, the proper attitude and knowledge are required.

Being distinctive matters

Even while having the ideal body is believed to be the key, it is insufficient. It doesn't matter much at all. Even with the most attractive body, one would occasionally fall short of expectations. The audience and the camera are the main factors taken into account. You may have an advantage if a good image is projected when the lenses are attempting to project positively. Additionally, you must have a certain quality that makes you stand out from the crowd. People have achieved success long before they entered the modeling industry, only to find that their appearance is unchanged. Therefore, it's crucial that you stand out from the crowd and have something to be proud of even when you're surrounded by other models.

Attend to the details

In the fitness sector, you would essentially notice that the unimportant things you previously believed did not matter are actually equally crucial to everything else. You must look after your own needs. Simple, seemingly insignificant details like your nails would be incredibly important. One key word in the fitness industry is loving and caring for one's body.

There are numerous basic and minor talents that are vital. Correct taste, fashionable clothing, decent grooming, and good hygiene are important. positive attitude and

Health And Fitness- Make It The Choice

Every fitness model should have attitude. This is mostly due to the fact that as you faced the camera and the crowd, everything about you would be sent to them and entirely define you. Your soul and body would then combine when you got there.

If you have the appropriate attitude and the conviction that you are on the right path, the glamorous and exciting world of modeling will be waiting for you.

Without a question, maintaining good health and fitness is a crucial aspect of being a person. The health of oneself and one's family must be taken seriously.

The health of every member of your family is something you value equally with your own. When given the opportunity, many people read articles on family fitness and family health precisely for this reason. About fitness and health, there are numerous books, articles, periodicals, emails, e-books, and newspapers. The majority of reading materials appear to be unclear, overly detailed, excessively lengthy, overly serious, and occasionally too complicated. These materials, however, are exactly what you need to know.

Unused information isn't quite as bad as useless information. This means that no matter how many books you find on fitness and health, they are useless unless they are used effectively. You can find all the health and fitness information you need. Various writers, experts or even trainers have differing things being expressed. Hence you might start sooner by working upon your family health and fitness straight away.

Below are few basic techniques which would assist you in your quest to acquire a fit and healthy family life.

1. Eat only healthy diet

You need to grasp what is meant by a healthy diet. Parents must set adequate examples to their children about intake of healthful food. Your kids would surely adopt a similar eating pattern if they witness you consuming healthy stuff. You are not required to become an expert in food preparation. You can feed your family nutritious food every day if you have a little imagination in the kitchen and some knowledge of various food types.

2. Include proteins

Right from breakfast to dinner, ensure to take meals high in proteins. It could include turkey, red meat, eggs, chicken, fish or cottage cheese. Proteins are necessary in your body as they

continue to build muscle. As it is the key, this is necessary once more for fantastic health and fitness.

3. Limit saturated fat intake.

Fats could be bad for the body. However, if you incorporate healthy fats in your diet, you will be moving toward a fit and healthy physique. Always keep a safe distance from saturated fat because it may be dangerous.

4. Regular exercise

One needs to understand the importance of everyday exercise. You might also concentrate on creating a family exercise schedule, encouraging kids to follow suit so they can learn the benefits of regular exercise. Start with a schedule that calls for two hours of exercise per day over the course of five days. Try as many crunches as you can and make sure to perform them correctly. Teach your kids a few basic crunches so they can practice them alone while you perform a few more challenging ones.

5. Walk the talk

Talk to your family as a whole and to your kids in particular. Everyone must be aware of the proper motives for exercising and achieving particular objectives. Your family will eventually support you when they come to understand your aims and see that you are committed and dedicated.

The trick is to get your entire family on board with your exercise plan. The secret would be realized only when everyone work out together. You don't need to think too much about books, papers, etc. because you already know what the necessary fitness exercises are. If you take immediate action, you'll see that your family is leading a fit and healthy lifestyle. Your efforts may help your family avoid health issues in the future.

You've heard that stretching is something you ought to do ever since you were a young child. No matter if you are just getting ready for the day or are planning a five-mile run, stretching is a need, you have been taught. This is actually extremely true, in my opinion. Although most people would claim to understand the need of stretching, most are unaware of its benefits. Of again, it's also possible that most people don't do it. You'll better appreciate why stretching is necessary if you are aware of what occurs during the process.

The Science first

The muscular fibers are extended when you stretch your muscles. They are removed. However, some of those fibers do maintain their usual, or resting, size. By fully stretching the muscle, you prevent it from becoming harmed or otherwise impaired when it is in use. Because your muscles are at rest when your body is, they are not fully prepared for use. The muscles get shorter and tighter the longer they are at rest.

You will quickly realize that you need full range of motion for your muscles if you think about what you will be using them for. There are issues, for instance, if you need to extend your leg muscles in order to run but they aren't fully extended. First, the muscles are overly contracted, which prevents full function. Second, if you pull the muscles too far, they could become injured because they are tight.

You can see how crucial it is that you take some time to stretch. You restrict what your body is capable of by failing to do this. If you attempt to stretch those muscles past their current state, you run a serious risk of injury. The objective is to provide yourself muscles that are entirely flexible, nimble, even, and capable of assisting you in effectively completing your activities. To do this, you must consider adding a stretching workout to your day. You should examine what stretching may do to increase your body's abilities as well.

Stretching And Weight Loss

Stretching should be done as part of your weight loss regimen. Nothing compares to the dull aching that runs through your body as you begin weight reduction activities. Exercise is difficult and exhausting on both your body and mind if you are even a little overweight. Stretching before and after every workout is one approach to improve the effects that exercise has on your body. Stretching by itself won't help you lose weight, but it will get your body ready for everything that will come next. That is the thing you need to think about.

Getting Stretched

Stretching should be done before to beginning your workout. Work on extending every muscle group and rotating every joint starting at the top of your body. Allow your body to truly feel the stretching as you do this while remaining calm. When this occurs, your body will be completely awakened and ready to benefit fully from the upcoming workout. Additionally, you'll be able to give your body the finest defense against harm in the future. You can start your workout after safely, slowly, and actively stretching every muscle in your body.

Following Your Workout

Once your workout is through, it's time to start stretching once more. Why should you extend right now? Before working out, stretching helps your body get ready and prevents injuries. By stretching now, you will help your body start repairing your muscles and make tomorrow's soreness less severe. By stretching right away, you give your body a chance to cool down and adjust to the fact that your workout is already beginning to repair.

You may feel fantastic before, during, and after your workout by stretching in this way. By stretching before your workout, you not only get more out of it but also prevent yourself from getting hurt. This enables you to get the most all-around effective workout possible. Therefore, you won't be too sore to exercise tomorrow. All of this results in the ability to lose weight more quickly and successfully.

Understanding What Stretching Is

Stretching is a common workout that is required to do and is particularly significant when it comes to physical fitness. The danger of injury and range-of-motion loss are likely to be factors for those who do not stretch adequately. Stretching has a very straightforward purpose.

The range of motion of the joint will be somewhat expanded by giving the muscle a stretch. People will exert force and strain on the affected part of the muscle in order to extend it. During this time, the muscle is also strengthened. The essential task can be performed more effectively by the muscles.

When It's Required

Stretching is not always essential. In reality, a lot of people will admit that they simply avoid doing it and don't get hurt. But whenever you want to conduct physically hard workouts, the majority of sportsmen and medical professionals will advise some kind of stretching. For instance, the situations where your body must be flexible and extended may be the best occasions to use stretching techniques on them. The body needs to have an increased range of motion for activities like long distance running, acrobatics, martial arts, and even ballet in order to perform more than it typically would. Without this stretching, the body's capabilities are severely constrained.

To prevent being hurt

The body's capacity to prevent injury is increased as another benefit of stretching. Stretching can help keep your muscles, ligaments, tendons, and other parts of your body from being hurt. Stretching makes the muscles more elastic, which explains why this is the case. In the higher ranges of motion you will utilize it in as it grows more elastic, it lessens the stretch reflex that could otherwise result in an injury to you.

Stretching is something that you should do because it can both improve your performance and help you avoid injury. You might not be able to do as well with the kinds of activities you're looking for if you don't stretch enough. Stretching properly is practically necessary for safety as well.

What Is Static Stretching?

Stretching comes in a variety of forms, including static stretching. You will stretch gently and only using your specific muscles during this form of stretching. As you are aware, stretching is a crucial component of getting ready for your workout. You must perform these warm-up exercises if you want to have the complete range of motion necessary to perform the workout or physically demanding activity. But you also need to stretch out after you work out. Static stretching is the ideal kind of cool-down stretching.

Why Does It Matter?

One muscle at a time is what one static stretching technique does to your body. Additionally called passive stretching. The methods used are smoother and simpler than other stretching techniques, as the name suggests. This makes it the ideal form of exercise to do after a workout or a few miles of jogging. You should incorporate static stretching into your workout routine as an after-workout stretch.

During a static stretch, you will comfortably stretch your muscle. You'll do this to the level that is comfortable for you to move it. By going just as far as you can comfortably go, you allow the muscle to begin to relax. Start by straightening the arm or leg until it is no longer possible to do so comfortably. For twenty to thirty seconds, maintain your position.

You are securely stretching your muscles by performing the stretches in this manner. You're doing it slow and gradually allowing your muscles to extend further. In a lot of respects, static stretching is the kind of stretching that is seen as the most secure.

Static stretching is the best option for cool-down activities, despite the fact that it is insufficient for a warm-up activity. Only perform a few light static stretches if you choose to throughout your warm-up exercises. The stretch could be too strong for a muscle that is cold. However, it is considerably simpler to do and offers more advantages for a warm or used muscle.

You can efficiently cool down by finishing your workout with static stretches. It is also a terrific technique to maintain your muscles agile and even assists to lessen the soreness you'll feel the next day after your workout.

Ballistic Stretching

Ballistic stretching is sometimes called active stretching. In this sort of stretching, you don't only extended the muscle outwards. Instead, you are engaging in a lengthier and more intricate stretch. If you have never stretched before, you should work on learning a few stretching techniques that incorporate ballistic stretching techniques. In fact, you should incorporate this kind of stretching into your exercise routine. Ballistic stretching allows for the perfect warm up before you exercise. For that reason, everyone that will do any type of hard or semi challenging exercise will need to concentrate on incorporating ballistic stretching into their training regimen as their way for warming up.

What Happens?

You will employ motion and momentum together with ballistic stretching to fully lengthen your muscles. Your body will go through a series of motions during this kind of stretching in order to urge muscles to be more flexible for your upcoming routine or exercise. You'll use a particular kind of swift movements that will result in a stretch position.

The kind of ballistic stretches you choose should be properly thought out and somewhat relevant to the kind of activity you'll be performing after the stretches. You won't utilize heavy ballistic stretches to warm up when you include them in your workout. If not, you run the risk of getting hurt.

For one light ballistic type of stretch, do the following. Stand with your arms at your side. Relax. Now, lengthen each of your joints after first flexing them. After that, carefully rotate each joint. You can use your feet, hips, toes, shoulders, wrists, elbows, fingers, ankles, knees, shoulders, and trunk to do this. If you want to, you can repeat them.

By giving your body particular ballistic stretching workouts, you enable your body to get used to doing the tasks that will later require more power from it. It can be a really effective warm-up to get your body ready to go and perform what you want it to. You run the danger of hurting those joints if you don't provide this kind of stretching. Try to incorporate some of these ballistic stretching exercises before you begin in addition to your regular workout. This will increase the workout's effectiveness even further.

You understand the value of maintaining a healthy weight as a runner. Stretching should be a part of staying in shape. Despite the fact that you might not be aware of it, you should spend a few minutes learning about and practicing stretches. No matter if you are a new runner or someone that has been running for years, adding stretches into your workout can and will allow you to do more, accomplish better goals and it will allow you to successfully accomplish tasks in a more complete manner. It also will prevent you from injury in some circumstances.

Running: It's A Physical Test

Your body tenses and you can feel your adrenaline pounding as you approach the starting line for your race. Your body is ready to go if you were able to warm up. It is prepared to offer you its all straight away when the time arrives to start the race. However, if you haven't done enough warm-up stretches, your body will start out slowly and have trouble with the initial steps as it starts to loosen up. Slowly, your muscles begin to stretch and your range of motion is more. You may feel your legs begin to loosen.

What's wrong with waiting for this to happen instead of extending in the first place? The bottom line is what you want and need from your body. If you just consider your legs, for example, you need that first stride over the line to be the best step it can be. You need to make sure that everything that happens during this event is something that can aid you to power through your training and race from the start to the finish. You've fallen further behind than you should have by preventing your body from giving it its best right away.

Many runners commit the error of not stretching before they begin their run on the track. This can be very problematic and frequently leads to you losing both your balance and your position at the finish line. If you allow yourself the type of stretches that will prepare your body for that run, the end result is that you will actually succeed, better than before.

<u>Body Building And Stretching</u>

You must stretch if you are bodybuilding. It makes no difference whether you are engaging in a minimal amount of muscle building or a full-on exercise program. You must include stretching in your training objectives. Although you might not yet be aware of the advantages of training, you will start to see them when you start incorporating it into your regular workouts. Learn why stretching and bodybuilding go hand in hand by taking a few minutes.

What It Does For You

Man or woman, stretching is a vital component of the process of working out. There are several things that it does for you in fact. It improves appearance, lengthens your muscles, and significantly contributes to the development of muscles that are lean and toned. It can help to enhance your fitness level and it will boost your general health as well. That's a lot to gain from just a few minutes of stretching. Of course, if you are at an event, it surely helps you to show off those muscles as well!

Stretching can help you warm up for your workout and will help you avoid overextension injuries overall by 50%. This is common knowledge in any athletic community, and it also applies to bodybuilding. You'll discover that stretching can also make you feel less sore after your workout in addition to giving you this kind of added support.

Stretching in a dynamic manner before your workout is recommended. To thoroughly prepare the body for what is to come, focus on each area separately. Install a cool-down stretching exercise as well after your workout. Stretching should be more static during this workout. This is the area where you will benefit the most in terms of recovery from an injury and relief from soreness the following day.

While bodybuilding is labor-intensive, it can have profound positive effects on your body. Make sure you are properly warmed up for the exercises you will be performing after your warm up by looking at a variety of stretching techniques. You will find this to be an excellent warm up and cool down to virtually any body building workout you may do.

Stretching was mentioned by your elementary school gym teacher, yes, but why should you do it now? You are healthy. Both before and after your workout, you feel absolutely comfortable. So, what is it that you may possible get from a few simple and monotonous stretches? Unfortunately, this mindset puts you at risk and could lead to unfortunate events. In some cases, athletes have even claimed that stretching reduces their risk of injury from overextending by 50% compared to not stretching. It is worth the few extra minutes to make this happen.

Here are some benefits of stretching before and after your workout or physical activity.

• Stretching makes your body more flexible. This flexibility is necessary to achieve a full range of motion for the physical challenge or workout you intend to subject your body to.

• Stretching aids in reducing soreness following exercise. You can minimize the dull discomfort that indicates you had a solid workout. Stretching actually encourages healthy muscle growth and helps your muscles get ready for a quicker recovery.

• Stretching also aids in the prevention of posture issues.

Your body can move more easily and productively if it has more, well-developed muscles.

• Stretching will broaden your range of motion, enabling you to advance more quickly.

• Stretching maintains the health of your muscles not just now, but well after your active years of exercise.

• You reduce the risk of injury when you do stretching exercises that are appropriate for the activity that you will be doing before you do it. Much fewer over extensions actually occur.

• Stretching promotes the growth of muscles that are bigger, better able to meet your needs, and that burn fat more quickly than muscles that don't. You acquire superior quality muscles

then without stretching.
• Stretching also improves the appearance of your muscles. Without stretching, they appear more attractive, toned, and natural.

Stretching provides many benefits for anyone who needs to exercise. Regardless of whether you are exercising because you want to get in shape, want to reduce weight, or just because you want to run a 5 mile run the following week. Including it in your workouts can help you develop into a well-muscled machine.

When Is The Right Time For Stretching?

Right, stretching is a regular element of exercise. One of the biggest mistakes people make is not knowing when to stretch if something isn't already the case but you're trying to change it. It makes no difference if you want to warm up for a bodybuilding workout, a ballet performance, or a marathon. You must learn when it is appropriate to stretch. This will contribute to giving you the overall health advantages necessary for maximum effectiveness.

Before Extending

Know when to stretch to offer yourself the best chance to get the most from your workout. Start with a little warm-up or exercise before you start. Do this by using the treadmill's low intensity level for around 10 minutes. Alternately, use the exercise bike for a short while. Simply getting the blood pumping and the muscles moving is the main objective here.

Why do you need to stretch after warming up? That has an easy solution. The muscles in your body are said to be warm if they have been used at all. However, if you start stretching straight away, you don't allow them enough time to "wake up," as it were. Instead, spend a short time warming up on the bike at a low effort. Finally, stretch. Stretching will become easier as a result, and it will also be better for you overall. After doing this, continue with the rest of your workout. Now, you'll be able to enter the groove with ease and lessen the chance of getting hurt.

Stretch continuously

However, stretching is not just for after a workout. Every day, you should stretch to benefit your body. This indicates that you should exercise for ten to fifteen minutes every day. You will notice that your general health benefits and your workout days will rise if you do this just three to four times each week.

Also crucial immediately following your workout is stretching. After the workouts, performing certain activities is the appropriate cool-down. It keeps your muscles active while still enabling them to easily maintain warmth and prevent injuries. Yes, feel free to include stretching in your routines. Do them prior to working out, afterward, and even on your days off. With each routine you perform, you'll observe progress.

You can improve your entire health and well-being by stretching. Stretching at various intensities should be incorporated into your tough training routine. Stretching promotes muscular growth and enables your muscles to work as efficiently as possible for you without risking injury. Stretching can help you achieve the finest overall workout possible when it comes to getting in a solid workout.

What Do You Do, though?

Depending on the type of exercise you intend to undertake after each stretch, each type is likely to alter slightly, but there are a few key ideas you should grasp and master right away. You should always incorporate static stretching into your workout, for instance. Some people do this prior to workouts and others after. Your muscles can be slowly and softly stretched while everything is under control by using static stretching. This makes it possible for your body to benefit you overall without running the risk of becoming damaged.

Additionally, make sure you are correctly stretching each muscle group. The proper technique involves stretching the opposing muscle groups. Stretch your quads and hamstrings, for instance, as well as your triceps and biceps. Never perform just one since doing so will throw your muscles out of balance, increasing your risk of injury and reducing the amount of flexibility you may achieve from your entire stretch.

Don't overextend yourself when it's time to stretch. You shouldn't immediately extend your muscles to their maximum length. Instead, lengthen your muscle and gradually extend it further at a time. This will enable you to stretch the muscle gradually, reducing the risk of harm from stretching. You should take about 30 seconds to reach the full stretch, after which you can hold it for another 30 seconds.

To get the benefits from stretching that you need for your particular activity, you must learn how to stretch properly. While running, stretching your arms won't be as effective as stretching your legs. By including stretching in your total workout in this way, you will encourage your body to benefit as much as it can from the exercise you intend to accomplish.

24 Hours Fitness Center

Imagine having a muscular, attractive body. Imagine that you achieved that status by having fun and making new friends when most businesses are closed. Consider yourself to be robust and healthy, free from disease, and bursting with enthusiasm.

Do you think this is a pipe dream? Okay, so it's not.

Although they might be in your dreams, those pictures are real. How? Through a regular routine of exercise at a 24 Hour Fitness Centers.

All of these opportunities are available at 24 Hour Fitness Centers. That's how they become the greatest private fitness chain in the world.

Millions of individuals utilize 24 Hour Fitness Centers every day, at any time of the day, to achieve a beautiful, healthy physique and enhance their quality of life.

For people of diverse backgrounds from across the world, the 24 Hour Fitness Center has become a home away from home because of its flexible scheduling options, selection of top-notch equipment, and classes.

There are many of people with full schedules who

understand the value of scheduling a daily workout or specialized fitness class, even if it's late at night.

The schedules for group exercise classes are flexible and practical. Exercise equipment comes in a wide variety and is widely available. The knowledgeable staff is supportive and helpful. The importance of 24 hour fitness centers in helping people live richer, healthier lives and develop upbeat, enthusiastic outlooks cannot be overstated.

The instructors at 24 Hour Fitness Center think their work helps much more than just keep individuals physically fit and healthy. They'll tell you that those who take classes or receive personal instruction acquire better self-confidence and determination. They play a bigger role in society as a whole as their appearance and abilities advance.

The 24 Hour Fitness Center's staff members are committed to assisting their clients in developing a strong, fit body, excellent health, and a balanced lifestyle. They recognize that dedication and perseverance are essential elements of a healthy lifestyle and that expensive equipment cannot motivate these qualities on its own. They provide all of their clients with individualized support and inspiration.

And as many of us have learned, even modest success can have a big impact. Customers become more motivated and dedicated to regular exercise as their muscles become more toned, their flexibility and agility improves, and they start to feel better overall. Instructors emphasize that the amount of work students put into their exercise routine will directly correlate to their ability to achieve a beautiful figure and good health.

The quality of the equipment and facility, the convenience and flexibility of operation hours and practices, and personal expert support have made 24 Hour Fitness Center the most popular source for fitness aficionados worldwide.

Whether they're members for life or working on a short-term improvement plan, experienced fitness fanatics or anxious newbies, 24 Hour Fitness Center clients know they'll get high quality and dependable care when they make 24 Hour Fitness Center their home away from home.

When looking for a gym or health club in the future, consider 24 Hour Fitness Center. You'll be happy that you did!

24 Hour Fitness Centers And Clubs

A quality gym or fitness club may provide you with a number of tools and services to help you achieve your goals if you want to have and maintain a healthy, well-toned body. But keep in mind that not all health clubs are created equal.

You want a health club that has more motivation than just making money. So that you experience positive outcomes as soon as possible, it should be fully committed to health and excellent service. A knowledgeable, experienced staff should be there to assist you with your workouts and demonstrate how to utilize any new equipment. Additionally, it ought to provide a range of courses that concentrate on various facets of health and fitness. Another essential aspect you should search for is a trained dietician on staff.

You may rely on 24 Hour Fitness, which offers five different types of clubs to match your specific demands. From basketball and volleyball to saunas and spas, the Ultra Sport club has all the amenities and is set up for any form of workout you can think of. Even your rock climbing skills can be improved. You won't need to hire a babysitter because there is a kids' club, and there is a full juice bar for dietary wellness. You can go to a tanning booth or have a nice massage after your workout. The Super Sport Clubs at 24

Hour Fitness have many of the same features but no massage or rock climbing. The Sport Club does not provide tanning, just as the Super Sport. Weight training, aerobic exercises, sauna, steam room, and a kids' club are the main components of an active club. The Fitlite club also provides a variety of group classes and a thorough cardio workout.

With more than 385 clubs and having been in business since 1983, 24 Hour Fitness is the largest privately owned and run fitness center network in the world. They've employed competent nutritionists to supplement working out with outstanding advice on the foods you should - and shouldn't - eat for years in addition to maintaining a knowledgeable team to assist their clients in getting the most out of their exercise programs.

A major letdown and a waste of time and money is joining a new club only to discover that it lacks adequate facilities and equipment options. 24 Hour Fitness will not let you down. Modern fitness equipment is kept up to date for all workout requirements. You won't ever have to stop working out because the equipment broke down or wait for a machine to become available in order to obtain the exercise you require.

In order to help you learn new skills and have fun with your friends at the same time, they provide group classes and team sports facilities. Numerous types of exercise are covered in 24 Hour Fitness programs, including pilates, strength training, cardiovascular exercises, yoga, and water exercises. Over 7000 experts make up their global teacher staff, and 24 Hour Fitness keeps them up to date with the newest methods by providing in-house training for Group Trainers.

At 24 Hour Fitness, you have a variety of membership options to fit your schedule and your budget. Three separate one-club alternatives offer savings, terrific workouts, and short-term fitness programs, while four different all-club membership types grant you access to facilities all around the world.

Travelers should take use of the Passport Program, which allows you to use other private fitness facilities as part of your 24 Hour Fitness membership as they have locations all over the world. To receive a fantastic workout at any Passport Program member's facility, all you need is your 24 Hour Fitness Passport Program ID and a fair charge.

When 24 Hour Fitness partnered with five internationally renowned athletes in 2000, they took a risky step toward promoting fitness and transforming it into a way of life for all of us. These sports superstars serve as role models and tangible examples of the virtues that 24 Hour Fitness promotes (determination, hard work, tenacity, and a positive attitude). In order to promote 24 Hour Fitness and promote people's health, Lance Armstrong, Shaquille O'Neal, Magic

Johnson, Andre Agassi, and Jackie Chan all agreed to join forces.

In 2004, 24 Hour Fitness became the first fitness facility to officially sponsor a U.S. Olympic team, improving Olympic Training Centers all around the nation and providing funds to help athletes pursue their goals of competing in the Olympics. Their dedication to wellness is evident.

At 24 Hour Fitness, working out will be enjoyable, simple, and individually satisfying. You'll discover a broad variety of exercise options and tools, comprehensive modern facilities and amenities, and a seasoned team to assist you in meeting your objectives quickly.

It's your responsibility to look into 24 Hour Fitness if you're looking for a health club.

Need An Inexpensive Lifecycle Elliptical Trainer?

Today, lifecycle elliptical trainers are offered for purchase in almost all fitness equipment stores. It should come as no surprise that Lifecycle is a well-known, premium brand of elliptical trainers, cycles, and treadmills. However, you have probably discovered that lifecycle elliptical trainers are not inexpensive if you have sought for them on sale. Simply said, you won't find a brand-new Lifecycle elliptical trainer for sale in discount stores today. However, you may be able to discover a lifecycle elliptical trainer for sale at a lower cost than you would for a brand-new one.

Contacting gyms and training facilities for a used equipment is one way to get good lifetime elliptical trainers for sale at reduced prices. You might be able to locate a decent deal on a Lifecycle elliptical trainer for sale through these facilities' sales office as they frequently upgrade their equipment. You might be able to purchase a lifetime elliptical trainer through their leasing businesses since they regularly lease workout equipment. They also replace used equipment, and their sales offices might have what you're looking for.

Searching for refurbished lifecycle elliptical trainers for sale at fitness equipment repair shops or at manufacturer's outlets is a fantastic choice. Customers frequently exchange new equipment for a different model when it malfunctions. The vendor then restores the device and offers it for sale at a substantial discount. Refurbished equipment is just as reliable and affordable as new equipment. In order to get an excellent machine and save money, looking for a lifecycle elliptical trainer for sale at a refurbish discount is a wonderful idea. Another benefit of a refurbished machine can be the warranty. You might be able to receive limited coverage in case you run into issues, albeit it might be shorter than the warranty that was included with the equipment when it was bought new. For a machine that is as good as new, you are still spending significantly less.

If you're a roving shopper, there are probably a lot of auctions, flea markets, yard sales, and garage sales where you can locate lifecycle elliptical trainers for sale. Whether we like to admit it or not, people frequently purchase new fitness equipment but only use it for a few challenging exercises before giving up. Even a Lifecycle elliptical trainer can be available for purchase at an estate auction. On a lifecycle elliptical trainer for sale by private sellers, you should be able to obtain a great deal and save a ton of cash. But take care. To ensure you purchase a Lifecycle elliptical trainer for sale that is functional and has all of its parts, you must meticulously inspect the equipment. Probably, you won't be able to the lifecycle elliptical trainers for sale here come with a warranty. You will, however, receive a fantastic piece of equipment at an extraordinary bargain if the unit functions well.

Any way you choose to look for a lifecycle elliptical trainer for sale, you may save money and purchase this premium item. When you can find a terrific deal, it's worth the time and effort to perform a comprehensive search. You can obtain a lifetime elliptical trainer for a healthy life from a gym, the company that makes its equipment, a refurbished, or a former user.

Taking A New Look At Diet And Fitness

For the majority of us, health and fitness have risen in importance over the past few decades. Some people are drawn to the attention that comes with having a killer body. Others desire flawless abs, a smaller waist, or biceps that are protruding. This movement has led to an increase in the number of gyms, health clubs, spas, and personal trainers.

Television is flooded with advertisements for workout regimens, weight reduction aids, and equipment, making it difficult to believe you're the only person watching who isn't working on your body. A healthy, fulfilling existence is actually a part of having the ideal body.

A balanced diet and a healthy lifestyle are necessary for true health. Diet for fitness gives us the nutrition and energy we need to repair worn-out muscles and keep our energy levels up and productive. Consider the following diet plans: Scarsdale, Atkins, South Beach, high-carb, low-fat, all-protein, sugar-free, and chocolate. There are plenty of appealing fad diets out there.

You might not know where to look for reliable, frank information about nutrition and health if you pay attention to ads and special programs that promote diets and weight loss plans. The majority of fad diets don't actually work and are definitely bad for your health. What can you do, then, to determine what is best and healthiest for you?

In actuality, there are only two types of diets: high-carb and high-fat. High-carb and heavy-fat diets emphasize the consumption of foods high in carbohydrates and fat, respectively. High-carb diets consume the glycogen in your muscles' and liver's stores for energy. You can use this glucose complex to get rapid energy for anaerobic workout.

The richest source of calories is fat, which has a calorie value that is more than twice as high as that of either carbohydrates or proteins. The body uses 24 calories to break down carbohydrates, whereas only three calories are needed to break down the same amount of fat.

Which is the best, then? Neither. Results can be obtained with any diet strategy as long as you stay to it. You can follow a low-carb, high-fat diet or a high-fat, low-carb diet. Simply avoid attempting both at once unless you want to put on weight.

However, decreasing fat shouldn't be the only goal of diets. A balanced, healthy diet helps people stay at a healthy weight and prevents weight gain. Only when the daily diet matches lifestyle, individual food choices, particular physical needs, and feeling satisfied with what you eat can make you achieve the desired weight loss. Really, there is only one diet that will be effective for you. That diet will keep you in shape, healthy, and content with who you are. And only you can follow that diet.

Three things should be kept in mind when dieting for fitness: moderation, variety, and balance. Make sure to organize your meals so that you never feel overly hungry or full at any point of the day. This could refer to one meal, three meals, or five meals. It depends on your physical requirements and timetable.

When you eat in moderation, you simply consume the number of calories necessary to satisfy you without adding extra calories that your body would only store as fat. Balance entails choosing a variety of foods from the fundamental food groups. It entails consuming the right proportions of proteins, carbs, fats, and fiber to maintain optimal bodily performance. Giving yourself enough options allows you to remain engaged in the things you eat. Eating the same foods over and over again is harmful as well as boring. You may ensure that you get the nutrition and variety you need by eating chicken one day and a salad the next.

Bottom line: Choosing a diet plan that will actually work is not your most essential option. What eating strategy will keep YOU in shape and healthy? It does not entail following a trendy diet for a few weeks or months before reverting to your previous routines. It entails making a well-balanced, wholesome diet your own, sticking with it for the rest of your life, and getting regular exercise.

One final piece of advise is to experiment. To keep your diet interesting and nourishing, try new foods. To gain a fresh twist on the tried-and-true, try different dishes. The future? Even learning to enjoy spinach is possible!

Exercise And Play

Many kids look worn out and ready for a sleep when they return following an afternoon of play. Play is a lot of labor for youngsters. Children's play involves more than just playing. It allows kids to develop physically, socially, and emotionally and aids in their development into responsible, successful people.

Busy parents may be tempted to assign their children household tasks and homework rather than letting them play outside or giving them a book or art supplies because of their employment and other adult duties. But parents must keep in mind how crucial play can be in preparing their kids to eventually participate in the adult world as mature, content individuals.

Both zoologists and anthropologists understand how crucial play is to the development of most mammal species' young. Physically and socially healthy development depends on play. Those who played as children, both by themselves and with others, tend to be the healthiest, most well-adjusted adults.

Play aids in our social and emotional growth in addition to helping us build fine motor skills and strong, healthy bones and muscles. Being a part of a close-knit team, playing organized games, and participating in organized sports all help us become more human and teach us how to interact with others. Play is crucial in the modern corporate environment to gain the abilities required to succeed professionally.

What do we learn through playing?

- how to read body language; - how to handle conflict; - how to appreciate nature; - how to express our thoughts to others; - how to use our imagination to come up with workable solutions.
- how to have pleasure in everyday pursuits and other people
- how to cooperate and share; - how to respect others' contributions; - how to contribute effectively to a team;

The act of playing is crucial to self-discovery. Play not only develops a physically healthy body but also teaches us our strengths and weaknesses. It teaches us how to restrain our animalistic human inclinations, such as hostility, rage, and violence. Through play, we pick up the language and traditions of our community and integrate ourselves into it. Play teaches us to use our imagination and creativity to achieve our objectives and address our issues. Play teaches us learn to comprehend the signals that our bodies convey to our brains. Subtle forms of communication include responding to signals, throwing a ball at a target, and using facial expressions. We discover how to decipher and convey such covert messages as we play. We may learn about the natural world and the environment by playing.

Play continues to pay off for us throughout our lives. Because we grew strong bones and muscles, our bodies are stronger and we have a higher quality of life. Because we learnt how to collaborate with others for beneficial outcomes through play, our minds are sharper and our social skills are better. Because we learnt to recognize our own needs as well as those of others, engage in negotiation, and settle disputes, we have a more well-rounded emotional and psychological makeup. Finally, we discovered how to manage stress through exercise and physical activity.

So the next time you see a full trash can or more grass than you would like, take a moment to think before you interrupt Sally or Sam's game. Keep in mind that play is an essential component of learning to function in the world. Even though they'll finish their responsibilities, they'll prioritize play in your home.

<u>Earn The Benefits Of Regular,
Moderate Exercise</u>

Which type of exercise, aerobic or anaerobic, do you prefer? Are you aware of the distinction? Does it affect anything? Actually, no. The terms "aerobic" and "anaerobic" refer to various methods that the body obtains energy during activity.

Exercise that is aerobic, or done with oxygen, uses oxygen to fuel metabolism, with fat burning serving as the primary energy source. Muscle tiredness is comparatively less common during this form of activity. Exercise that involves aerobics is mildly intense. Exercise that is performed anaerobically, or without oxygen, is more intense and depends on sources of energy other than oxygen for the muscles. The primary fuel source for anaerobic activity is sugar. In any case, fat is still burned.

Light exercise encourages cell renewal while clearing out the waste product lactic acid. There are a few factors to keep in mind in order to burn fat instead of sugar:

- Inhale deeply. Breathe in through your nostrils using your diaphragm and hold the breath for a few seconds. the mouth to exhale next.

- Workout at a comfortable intensity. Exercise at a 7 if a 10 requires excessive effort. While working out, you ought to be able to carry on a typical conversation. You can recharge your batteries and feel terrific by doing this for 45 minutes each day.

You may not have the time you believe you do to exercise, but you should. Your health and general well-being will benefit significantly more than it will take time to do. You won't require as much sleep as you used to because regular exercise boosts energy. Take a little break from your sleep at night to exercise. You'll benefit from it more.

Alternately, you may work out during your lunch hour as opposed to eating a large, fattening meal. Your efficiency will rise. You'll have increased energy and alertness. Additionally, the time you save from increased productivity can be used for those other crucial duties that you wouldn't sacrifice for exercise.

Rebounding, sometimes referred to as cellularise, is an excellent cardio workout. A rebounder is a small trampoline that allows users to bounce for great, impact-free exercise. When you have Tried it! Access to this kind of equipment It's an enjoyable workout for people of all ages and fitness levels, and it costs less than other training gear.

Use any break or time out to walk about and breathe deeply, whether or not you have access to a rebounder. Any form of exercise has several advantages. Your heart will get healthier, stronger, and bigger as a result. Your lungs will become stronger as a result of deep breathing. Exercise movements encourage appropriate blood flow to both your muscles and joints, hence lowering the possibility of developing joint pain. Additionally, studies show beneficial relationships between physical activity and overall health, which can help fend against practically every disease.

Many of us spend the majority of our waking hours bent over our desks, concentrating on the task at hand while typing. Our bodies also get stiff, exhausted, and overflowing with natural poisons as a result of this. The right kind of exercise cleanses the body and stimulates all of the internal organs, including the brain. It revitalizes the body and elevates mood.

Simply investing a little time in moderate exercise will pay off with lifelong advantages. When you commit to and stick with a regular fitness regimen, you'll live better, longer, and with more enjoyment.

Outdoor Exercise And Fitness

The value of fitness and exercise is being recognized by more and more people. Whether indoors or out, you'll witness people making an effort to improve and maintain their health. Exercise outside is a great method to enhance your health and have fun at the same time!

For those who can afford them and have the self-control to continue going once they have paid their membership fees, gyms are a great resource. For those with plenty of space and money, home gyms are efficient ways to exercise. While they are "seeing" and "being seen," sociable types can take care of their health by participating in sports and other organized activities.

But what about people who have simple lives and are content spending time with their children or dog, don't need or desire a gym's structure, can't afford pricey equipment, can't work out and converse at the same time, or don't enjoy competition? Are they eccentrics? No!

A easy and enjoyable approach to stay in shape and take in nature is to exercise outside.

Exercise outside doesn't cost much. There isn't much preparation necessary. And anyone can choose it as a healthy lifestyle option. Among the many advantages of exercising outside are:

- You don't need special tools to do it.

- you won't have to deal with boisterous individuals and crowded gyms

- You won't need to go far to get there.

- The air is clean, and you can feel the wind in your hair.

- There are no membership fees or down payments required.

- You don't need to wear that specific attire.

- You are not required to wear makeup

- You do receive plenty of sunlight and vitamin D for strong bones and healthy skin.

- You can perform it whenever and anywhere you want to.

Now that you know that exercising outside is a terrific method to remain in shape and live a healthy life, you may be wondering what to do when you go outside.

The following are seven well-liked outdoor activities that will offer you a wonderful work out and leave you feeling fatigued, hot, and fantastic!

* Lunges

Lunges are a fantastic outdoor workout that can be done in a variety of ways to target your hamstrings and lower body. This is how drop-knees are often done. Your knees should be at a 90-degree angle while you stand with your feet about three feet apart. Make sure your heel is flat on the floor and your knees are directly over the centers of your feet before bending your knees and lowering yourself back toward the ground. As you push through the front heel and take a step back to the beginning position, maintain a straight upper body. Keep your knees from locking. Simply keep going in a fluid motion.

* Push-ups

Push-ups, which are excellent for your upper body, come in a variety of forms, including conventional, broad, and close grips. They are the ideal outdoor exercise, and by switching up the three movements, you may target more muscle areas and improve your performance. Raise your hands for more comfortable movement. Raising your feet will provide greater resistance. Try clapping your hands while bouncing if you're feeling very bold. Beginning with a straight back and knees that are parallel to the floor. When your nose contacts the floor, slowly lower your body to the starting position before quickly pressing back up. As often as you can without being too stressed out, repeat.

* Squats

Squats are a simple exercise to perform outside that, when done correctly, have a ton of force. They are less powerful when carried out incorrectly. Squats can be performed standing, on one leg, with a wide stance, in a pile, or overhead. Your legs will start to feel fatigued as you complete repetitions. This is advantageous. They work wonders to build your thighs, butt, and hips. Place your feet evenly apart as you stand. Keep your stomach in and your back straight. Just behind your toes, place your knees. Squeeze your butt as you stand, and squat to chair height. Repeat.

Holding weights in your hands while squatting will give you a more intense workout.

* Step-ups

If done correctly, this may be a punishing outdoor workout. A bench can be used as your equipment. Step up and down, keeping your back straight and your head held high, is all that is required. Back away from the platform (weights in hand for more power). As you step into the step, place your right foot on the bench and shift your weight to the heel. Just use your right leg; use your left leg simply to maintain balance. Step back gradually. Before moving to your left leg, perform this at least 10 times with your right leg.

* Chin-ups

Likewise called pull-ups. Use a piece of playground equipment or a tree limb. Take an overhand grip on the pull-up bar. Just wider than your shoulders, your grip should be. Leave your body as high as you can and gradually revert to your starting posture (don't fall). As many times as you can, repeat the movement. The sweat will start to flow after this outdoor workout!

* Sprints uphill

Those who can run a 100-meter dash should only attempt this. The simplest outdoor exercise is to find a hillside and sprint as quickly as you can up it. Go down and do it again.

* A duck trots

For those who are unafraid! This easy-but-difficult outdoor exercise will build your stamina and leg strength. Just lower yourself into a squat until your thighs are parallel to the ground. Then, take ten steps back while still in that position. As many times as you can (which probably won't be many).

Exercise outside is beneficial for your health. If done correctly, these outdoor exercises will provide you with advantages on par with—if not better than—those obtained from using the most costly equipment available in the poshest gym in town. You may recall how wonderful it is to be outside, rain or shine, taking in the fresh air and listening to the birds sing by engaging in outdoor activity. So, get started! Try some exercise outside right away!

Build The Best Home Gym At Fitness Depot

A healthy, attractive physique is a fit, well-toned body. Statistics indicate that diabetes, obesity, and other chronic diseases are on the rise despite all the fanfare. The best thing you can do for yourself and your family is to have and adhere to a thorough health plan. A balanced diet and regular exercise will both be part of this strategy. One store where you can get everything you need to develop a robust, healthy body and a sharper mind is Fitness Depot.

Nowadays, working out at the gym is a common activity. However, despite paying fees and dues, many people fail to consistently visit the gym. They might not have time to get to the gym. They can also have obligations, such as children, that demand their attention and make going to the gym a luxury. Others simply stop utilizing the gym because they no longer find it interesting. And those of us who are shy wouldn't even enter a gym for fear of seeming foolish.

The solution to this issue is as easy as buying home gym equipment and working out whenever you can in a setting where you can be easily reached in an emergency. There are many different types of home gym equipment and vendors all across the nation who can offer quality fitness equipment at fair prices that will fulfill your needs and keep you in shape.

Fitness Depot is a well-known and highly recommended provider for top-notch home exercise gear. It is the biggest retailer of fitness equipment in Canada, and it has locations across the country.

You may believe that establishing a home gym is a pricey endeavor, and in some ways, you're correct. You genuinely do get what you pay for. You'll likely need to invest in a number of different machines to target various body parts if you want to follow a well-rounded fitness regimen and get a full-body workout. Fitness Depot's professionals can assist you in determining your requirements and choosing the ideal exercise equipment for your particular circumstance.

The first Fitness Depot was established in 1993 by Marc Dubois and Edwin Cameron, and it was situated at 40 Ronson Drive in Toronto. Fitness Depot quickly became one of the most well-liked sources for fitness equipment thanks to consistent sales, dependable fitness equipment, and dependable support. in its initial

There are 36 locations around Canada, including one in Toronto that is still open. Major American cities are home to Fitness Depot locations as well.

Fitness Depot carries devices to help you acquire cardiovascular workout, strength training, even boxing. It offers a wide choice of fitness equipment brands and designs. There are treadmills, elliptical trainers, exercise cycles, home gyms, power blocks, rowing machines, steppers, and inversion beds available. For each training style, you can choose from a selection of accessories.

A trip to the neighborhood Fitness Depot will be rewarding if you want to create the ideal home gym that blends the comfort of home with the expert, high-quality exercise found in commercial gyms. You can be guaranteed to receive excellent guidance, first-rate support, and the ideal workout equipment for your requirements. Purchasing a home gym is an investment in your quality of life, health, and lean, trim appearance. Profit from the top-notch fitness equipment that Fitness Depot offers at affordable pricing. You'll be happy that you did

Health And Fitness For Singles

Living alone is wonderful! You are the one in charge. You have the freedom to act whenever you wish. Numerous dates. numerous parties. Numerous times!

That is the lie. However, if you're single, you know it's not quite that ideal. For singles, it might be difficult to make new friends, socialize outside of bars, and locate the ideal partner. Finding the proper acquaintances and the correct social opportunities can be difficult, perhaps even more so in the largest cities.

Additionally, singles must worry about maintaining their health and fitness, just like married people do. Did you know that it's possible to live a happy single life and a healthy lifestyle simultaneously? It exists. You can now enroll in a single exercise program created especially for independent, unburdened individuals. In the company of other singles, you can maintain your physical fitness and tone, meet physically fit friends, and share interests in a relaxed, cheerful environment.

You might even receive more exercise when you sign up for a single fitness program than you would otherwise. These services mix fitness regimens for singles with enjoyable activities you can partake in with other singles. Consider it.

Join other singles for team sports, swimming, cross-country mountain biking, and training routines.

If you believe that taking part in a single fitness program would be beneficial for you, you should look into the businesses and services that provide this kind of chance. They are neither escort or dating services. They are set up to provide opportunities for fitness so that working out would be more enjoyable and beneficial for singles' health. They understand that activities like biking or hiking alone can be monotonous and lonely. As a result, they gather singles in groups to share the experience.

You provide personal information to a single fitness program when you sign up so they can assist you select the exercise partners who are best for you. Your age, sexual orientation, preferred forms of exercise, and other personal preferences may be requested in order to locate the solution that best suits your requirements. They have a duty to pair you up with singles in your general age range and stage of life who share your interests, notably your fitness preferences.

You won't ever have to endure those monotonous, protracted workouts alone once you join a single fitness program. You'll never have to ride your bike alone along a rural road or walk a woodland trail alone, unless you want to. There will be those around you who share your desire to maintain your health. Even engaging in sports like boxing is possible within a single fitness regimen. They'll locate a sparring partner for you, and they'll go to the games.

Imagine the personal benefits of being able to engage in enjoyable social activities, undertake regular exercise, and keep a healthier, better-looking body. You might even cross paths with your ideal match! You'll already be aware of your shared interests. The relationship needs to be nurtured, and things should develop naturally after that. Nothing forcedly weird. There should be no bragging or lying to impress. When you realize that you are not at all alike, do not be disappointed.

You can start down a path that you can only fathom now with only one workout program. You'll have a wider group of friends that enjoy working out. Hours of social enjoyment will be had while you improve your health. Others will teach you something. You might even find the partner of your dreams!

Free Weights VS Machine exercise

You work out to improve your quality of life. However, even after an hour in the gym, your muscles still need to function efficiently for the following 23 hours without the aid of expensive machinery. No matter what kind of workout you're doing, your body's motion is referred to as its "range of motion." The exercise is more efficient the more challenging that range is.

You could have concerns regarding the most effective technique to accomplish your objectives, whether you're getting set to begin strength training for the first time or returning to a regular practice. Although beginners may feel more at ease with machine weights, they might not achieve the desired results. Machines may be more efficient for seasoned athletes who wish to concentrate on a particular muscle area. However, free weights are a tried-and-true technique that works regardless of size. With free weights, you might receive more value for your money, but you might also run a higher risk of injury.

Consider the traditional dumbbell bicep curl as an illustration. In order to perform this exercise, you must stand straight up with your palms facing forward and a dumbbell at either side of your body. You raise the dumbbell to shoulder height by flexing your biceps, then you do it as many times as you can.

When using a bicep curling machine, you sit with your arms braced on a pad, take hold of the handles in front of you, and move upward in a motion similar to how you did with the dumbbells.

For both workouts, the actions are practically the same. Your biceps are tightening. However, using the bicep curl machine while seated restricts shoulder motion. In the machine exercise, you use many forearm and finger muscles that you do not use when using dumbbells.

Whether you use free weights or a weight machine during weight training, the workout is essentially the same. You adhere to comparable practices with the same objectives. Machine weights, however, provide resistance, which modifies your exercise regimen in contrast to free weights. However, using a machine limits your versatility because it forces you to follow a set schedule with limited variations.

You have more freedom when using free weights, but it takes more effort to adjust the settings. You can alter your weights on a weight machine by flicking a switch!

People can be found on both sides of the argument. Many people think free weights are the best, while others say machine weights are more effective. While each has benefits and drawbacks, free weights have a longer history and have consistently shown impressive results.

Free weights have been used by bodybuilders for years with spectacular, competitive results. Any body builder you ask about machine weights will probably assume you're kidding.

Those who favor free weights claim that because they require more muscle activity than machine weights, they are more efficient. However, this does not imply that machine weights are a time and money waster. Machine weights aid in body stabilization and lower the risk of injuries.

Your decision about the sort of weights to use will be influenced by the goals you have for weightlifting as well as the location of your workouts. Both approaches work well and enhance your physique and health. While free weights require less room and give you greater flexibility in your exercises, they may also pose a higher risk of injury because of this. Machine weights are more expensive and less adaptable, but they are also more restrictive and take up more room.

Physical therapists claim that using both free weights and machine weights may be the most effective approach. The bottom line is that you must conduct the necessary study and base your choice on your own objectives and situation. You'll be able to choose the option that best suits your requirements by taking into account your time constraints, physical fitness goals, financial constraints, the accessibility of the facility, and other factors.

<u>Good Health And Fitness Is Easy And Free</u>

To increase your health and fitness, you don't need to acquire pricey equipment or join a gym. You can employ a variety of household objects in an efficient health and fitness regimen. Developing stronger muscles, increasing your strength, and increasing your endurance are all crucial to maintaining good health and fitness. Those can't be purchased, but you can earn them by participating regularly in a program that supports your fitness and excellent health. If you want to live a long, happy life, maintaining good health and fitness is a crucial objective.

You can receive all the exercise you need to improve both your physical and mental health if you adhere to these fundamental rules. Utilize them to create your own exercise and health plan.

1. Decide on an aerobic activity you enjoy and can perform either inside or outside. You can go hiking, running, strolling, playing tennis or soccer, or in-line skating. Make sure that whatever you do is vigorous and prolonged so that you can achieve a comprehensive body workout through cardiovascular conditioning or aerobic workouts. Ensure that your heart rate increases and remains elevated for at least

20 minutes.

2. To learn new exercises and have a leader to follow, use exercise videos. Today's market is flooded with intriguing and creative movies that offer a variety of exercises meant to boost your fitness and health. Someone has created a video to demonstrate how and keep you moving if you can think it up! These films provide a fantastic exercise and some decent enjoyment for a lot less money than a gym or equipment. Kickboxing, body rock, belly dancing, power yoga, and salsa dancing are a few examples outside of workout regimens tailored to particular body regions.

3. Get a solid workout and alter how you carry out tasks around the house. Use a push lawn mower as opposed to your power lawn mower. Completely vacuum the house. Clear the snow from the sidewalks and driveway. Carry your grocery bag or laundry basket several times up and down the stairs. As you go about your regular activities, wear weights around your ankles and wrists. You can make numerous minor changes to your fitness and health without even realizing it!

4. Play your preferred dance music and get up and move. Check your ballroom or hip-hop skills. No need to feel embarrassed because nobody is looking. Enjoy yourself. Take up contemporary dance. This is a fantastic method to burn some calories, enhance your fitness and health, and

reduce stress.

5. Plan social gatherings that are active. Invite your pals to play a game of touch football with you. Play a few hoops with the guys. Take up soccer. Invite a friend to join you for dancing classes. Take up racquetball. Build relationships and have a more active social life by exercising.

6. Plan any game-related events with your buddies. Kickball, football, basketball, soccer, and other sports may be involved. Other exercises that encourage muscle workouts through movement of the body are also an excellent choice.

7. Have the youngsters jump rope! This cardiovascular exercise is incredibly affordable and enjoyable!

8. Explore your neighborhood parks again. A lot of them include fitness trails you can follow that include suggested exercises, guidelines, and objectives. There is no longer any justification. You have everything in front of you. Simply start moving is all that is required.

There are countless things you can do to improve your health and fitness, and here are just a few ideas. As you read the recommendations, you could have come up with some of your own. Try them out.

Keep these pointers in mind before beginning any new training regimen:

* Never begin a workout session fully charged. When working out, it's crucial to warm up and cool down. You can't achieve ideal fitness and health in a single day. It takes time. Be tolerant. Start out gently and build up to a more strenuous regimen. Additionally, ALWAYS stretch both before and after exercising.

* Make an effort to exercise for at least 30 minutes each day. Don't stick to one activity for too long; switch things up. Keep it interesting, but carry on anyway. Achieving excellent health and fitness takes time. And maintaining a healthy lifestyle is a way of life, not a goal.

* Verify that you are utilizing the appropriate gear and attire for the exercise you have selected. Otherwise, you risk hurting yourself and delaying the steady advancement you desire. Consider the temperature both inside and outside when choosing your attire. Wear the appropriate clothing for the weather if you're working out outside. Additionally, you can continue your health and fitness regimen indoors if you are unable to exercise outside.

* Invite a pal to go with you. The buddy system works wonders for fitness and health programs. It increases the enjoyment of working out and gives you an opportunity to interact with others. Additionally, it increases the likelihood that you'll follow the plan over time. You might even incite

some constructive rivalry that will benefit you both!

* Switch it up. Alter the daily exercises you perform. Change how long you spend doing them. To avoid boredom and injury, keep your fitness and health regimen varied.

* Before beginning a new health and fitness program, always speak with your doctor to ensure that your goals are in line with your particular physical situation. You can't operate against your own body in this manner. Your doctor can suggest workouts that help strengthen you in the areas where you are weakest without causing serious or persistent issues.

* Exercise is just the beginning. A balanced, healthy diet will be a part of a thorough health and fitness regimen. Cut back on the sugar and up your intake of vitamins and minerals. Avoid going to the shop famished, and bring a well-thought-out list of tasty meals and plenty of variety.

These recommendations are simple to do, but for your health and fitness program to be successful, you must be disciplined and dedicated. You can have a healthy lifestyle and a toned body. You simply need to work for them. The advantages are priceless; you'll live a longer, happier, and higher-quality life.

Investing In A Home Gym

Everyone strives to look their best. You can see how self-conscious we've all become of our appearance and figure by taking a quick look at your television. But with all of the stresses and demands of daily life, it's simple to forget about our fitness and weight.

There never seems to be enough time for a consistent workout routine between work, kids, friends, and social obligations. Despite the abundance of gyms and fitness facilities, some may be out of reach. It might be too expensive to join or require too much of your time to be worth the hassle.

If you've ever felt frustrated about wanting to stay in shape but not having the time or money to join a gym, think about constructing your own home gym to get that gorgeous body and keep a fit, healthy body.

There are many different kinds of exercise gear that are excellent for use at home. Consider it. On the way to the gym, no more time is wasted in traffic. Your home gym is always open, so you don't have to worry about the time! You are not required to hire a babysitter or dress in expensive athletic attire. All you need to do is work out consistently for a lean, attractive body.

You might be wondering what equipment you'll need if you're thinking about buying a home gym. It might be worthwhile to join a gym for a brief period of time if you don't have much experience with fitness equipment and don't know someone who is knowledgeable in the field. Find out what will best suit your demands by looking at the equipment they use and speaking with their physical trainers. Try out various pieces of equipment to determine what you like and what suits you the best. Engage in some discussions with dependable members to learn what they believe about various brands and fashions. After learning some useful information, let your subscription lapse and begin creating your very own, custom-made home gym.

By concentrating on particular training forms or specific body goals, you can keep things straightforward and save money. By doing this, you'll be able to furnish your home gym with fewer distinct types of equipment and accessories. If money is not an issue, you can go all out and buy the toys. However, if you don't utilize them frequently, they can just end up becoming toys. As you acquire experience, our best advice is to start simple and build from a basic arrangement.

as well as physical stamina. If your home gym turns out to be as successful as we hope, you might also wish to add a room to the house.

You can learn more about the factors you should take into account while selecting the best home gym equipment from the conversation that follows.

Weight And Strength Training

Equipment for weight or strength training can be your best place to start if you want to develop strong muscles and a trim physique. Any excellent home gym must include weights. You might initially purchase free weights to determine if that is indeed what you want. Free weights can run you less than $50, but to get a solid workout you'll need a combination of them. smaller (9 kg) and 4.5 kg (10 pounds) weights that attach to a bar. You can add and remove various weights to perform a variety of exercises and to steadily increase your strength.

Traditional metal weights are available, however modern plastic weights could be simpler to handle and store. Many of the more recent weights can be adjusted to different weights without the need for extra purchases because they are filled with water or sand. Free weights are less effective for building hamstrings and calves.

Weight machines are useful for working on the biceps, quadriceps, and deltoids, among other muscular areas. They are more effective for working the muscles in the lower body, and using a machine reduces your risk of injury. However, using a weight machine in your home gym would take up more room. Simple resistance machines to adjustable multi-station weight stacks can range in price and configuration. You might spend hundreds to thousands of dollars to get a quality weight training machine for your home gym, depending on your goals and financial constraints.

stair climbing

A well-equipped home gym can start with these equipment. Stepping exercises help you build a tight butt and toned legs while providing a solid aerobic workout. The advantages for the heart are outstanding. Stepping can be done for as little money and as simply as utilizing a bench that is about 15" tall, or it can cost as much as a $80 to $150 stair stepper machine. More advanced stair stepper machines offer as many options as you want to pay for, including variable speeds and resistance levels, customizable speeds and pedal distances.

A excellent stair stepper will feature a heart rate monitor and digital readouts showing how many calories you've burned, how far you've come, and how quickly you've moved. The more advanced machines should cost roughly $2000.

These are just two of the many different equipment categories you may choose from for your home gym. We haven't included the more conventional and well-liked exercise equipment, such as rowing machines, treadmills, elliptical trainers, and bikes. Your home gym may have equipment with a wide range of costs and variable levels of quality.

Setting your personal fitness objectives is the first step to creating the ideal home gym. You'll be able to do your study and set a suitable budget for your home gym once you are clear on the outcomes you seek.

Consult experts, choose the appropriate gear, evaluate brands and pricing, prepare your area, and then enjoy creating your own home gym. One machine at a time is possible. You could stage a production of it. But you won't ever regret making the decision to live a better life and having a hot, healthy body.

The Importance Of Physical Fitness

A human body that is physically fit is one that can work without being too worn out. In other words, the body has a sufficient amount of energy reserves to work, play, and respond vigorously to physical demands. Your alertness, stamina, and strength, as well as your heart rate and blood pressure, are reliable measures of your physical fitness.

Your degree of coordination, flexibility, and agility also show your level of fitness beyond these fundamental indicators. Stress testing is a technique used by doctors to assess your physical fitness and identify issues by measuring your body's capacity to respond to continuous, intense physical demands.

One technique to train the body and increase physical fitness is through regular, planned exercise. Your body's capacity to handle everyday pressures can be maintained through regular, moderate exercise without putting your health at risk. But in order to increase vitality and sustain optimal physiological performance, the majority of people must start and maintain a regular, intense exercise routine

Seven Fitness Tips: Improving The Quality Of Life

1. Everyday exercise. You should perform activities that increase your heart rate, whether it be through a formal workout or through everyday activities. Aerobic exercises are a great method to increase your heart rate over time, but you may achieve the same result by performing household and office duties. Your heart rate might increase by making good decisions like walking instead of driving. Using a push lawn mower and using the stairs rather than the elevator are two other great ways to get daily exercise.

2. Consume more veggies and fruits. Fast food and processed meals are convenient, but they pose a risk to your health. Try to develop and maintain a healthy diet that includes lots of fruit and leafy green vegetables. They offer fiber, vital nutrients, and energy. Look for organic products that haven't been treated with pesticides or chemical fertilizers.

3. Work out using weights. Strength exercise improves endurance while constructing strong muscles and bones. Using hand-held dumbbells or a barbell can be an easy way to use weights during an exercise.

complex as cutting-edge weight training equipment. Weightlifting not only increases strength but also helps you slim down and get more chiseled muscles.

4. Consider circuit training. To get a more well-rounded workout, circuit training combines weight training with cardio workouts. You increase your cardiovascular fitness while also strengthening and toning your muscles. You perform a series of weightlifting exercises to gain strength quickly followed by aerobic workouts like squats, push-ups, trusts, or jumping jacks. After completing the cycle, you start over with the weights and complete the circuit a second time.

5. Get functional training. Functional training exercises imitate daily movements and activities and were first used to rehab patients with severe injuries so they may return to their professions and normal lives. It may include weight training to tone muscles or other exercises to increase coordination, flexibility, and agility, with an emphasis on the back and abdominal muscles.

6. Make sure to limber up. Resistance training that uses elastic strain to build and tone muscles through prolonged stretching is crucial as a warm-up before hard exercise. You may increase your mobility and range of motion by stretching, which also helps you become more flexible and strong. Your danger of getting hurt is also reduced. Stretching before and after arduous exercise reduces the risk of injury, raises heart rate, and increases muscle flexibility.

7. Drink plenty of water. Water is the most vital nutrient for life, and it makes up the majority of our bodies. We lose water and vital minerals during exercise that keep our muscles toned and our minds fresh and bright. Every person should consume at least two quarts of water each day, and those who are more active should consume even more. Four quarts of water per day should be consumed by anyone on a detox diet who is eliminating toxins and impurities from their systems. Coffee, tea, soda, and alcohol are some drinks that should not be drunk before or after exercise since they can dehydrate you. This is why a lot of athletic trainers and sports medicine specialists advise consuming so-called sports drinks. In addition to water, they also contain vital minerals that are lost during activity.

Although it's easy to overlook the value of these straightforward techniques in day-to-day living, they will assist keep your body in good shape and healthy. For a variety of reasons, people fail to incorporate regular exercise into their schedule. Perhaps they are under time pressure because of demands from work and family. Or perhaps they believe that in order to engage in healthful activity, they must join a gym. Perhaps they have an interest in

They have other interests and pastimes that they are unwilling to "give up" for fitness. Exercise unfortunately is not a luxury. It's important for preserving fitness and excellent health.

Reaching Your Body's Full Potential

- more illnesses as a result of decreased resistance - more accidents owing to poor agility and coordination
- increased risk of ill health brought on by being overweight or obese - increased susceptibility to some major diseases - increased physical and psychological stress (diabetes, heart disease, etc.)
- increased chance of requiring major surgery later in life

The fact is, we can't afford to skip our normal workouts. Maintaining a physically healthy physique is important for other reasons as well. It's a way to build and have a higher quality of life. Exercise helps you in many ways than simply physically. Your emotional equilibrium is enhanced, and you are better able to handle everyday challenges. It encourages constructive attitudes and changes negative thinking. It aids in the release of negative emotions like rage, minimizing the effects of ill-advised behavior. Boredom is alleviated, and you become a better, more lively companion for family and friends.

Put exercise and fitness at the top of your list the next time you organize and prioritize your day.

Exercise To Quit Smoking

Workout To Stop Smoking

When you decide to stop smoking, you'll need to adjust many aspects of your life. Smoking is incredibly difficult to stop since it is highly addictive. Numerous physiological changes will occur, and exercising is one approach to ensure success.

When you stop smoking, you'll need to create a new pattern and schedule to take the place of the numerous occasions when you used to light up. If you haven't been working out at a gym, you should start doing it because it will give your day a new dimension and help you temporarily forget about your former best friend.

Exercise to Change Your Routine

If a gym membership isn't realistic for you, you can still get a great workout to support your efforts to stop smoking. To get your pulse pumping and replace those early-morning old nicotine wake-up sticks, get up a little earlier and go for a little stroll. You may breathe in plenty of fresh air by making a run or job a regular part of your day. It's an excellent way to begin your new, smoke-free lifestyle.

Exercise doesn't have to be an intense workout if it's just one of your efforts to stop smoking. Being active, enhancing your health, and altering your routine are crucial. If you don't have the time or money for something more formal, simple exercising at home will do. It is simple to get going. Maintaining a new fitness routine tough. But if you're truly committed to giving up smoking, you need to make some significant adjustments. Regular exercise is a fantastic, healthier alternative that you should incorporate into your day.

Many had successful beginnings. You're going to stop using tobacco. You have confidence in your ability to complete it. You purchase exercise gear like gym attire, running shoes, and tights, and your first visit to the gym feels almost celebratory. When you stop smoking, things become challenging. Everything you bought, even the gym, doesn't seem as appealing. Your schedule is quite busy. You quickly decide against going to the gym. Soon you won't even be performing pushups in the bedroom. And then it takes place. You take hold of the cigarette.

You should aim to exercise early in the day to avoid the problems of exercise burn-out and jeopardizing your quit smoking plan. Many people like to workout in the evening, so it's okay if it fits your lifestyle. The majority of us, though, come to a complete standstill in the evening. Exercise is the last thing we want to do after a long day at work, taking the kids to activities, and attending to our adult obligations. But if you want to stop smoking, you must have the willpower to resist all temptations.

Your ability to resist temptation will improve as you feel better and have fewer cravings. You will have a far higher chance of sticking to your plan and actually altering your life if you workout before work or during lunch. So, if at all possible, schedule your workout in advance and commit to it.

Other Important Changes To Quit Smoking

Smokers have particular weaknesses; stimulants like caffeine, boredom, loneliness, and stress are all quit-trying smokers' triggers. Here are some ideas for handling certain situations:

* Steer clear of coffee and caffeinated drinks. replacing it with water. It won't make you crave cigarettes and is healthier for your health. Search for drinks devoid of caffeine. And until you get through those initial few trying days and weeks, stay away from chocolate.

* Don't fill unforeseen downtime. The greatest approach to prevent thoughts of smoking from entering your head is to stay active. Try to find something to do even at home to keep you occupied till the hunger passes. Dance while some music is playing. To give your room a fresh look and feel, rearrange your furniture or arrange your photographs. Get rid of any and all items in your home that make you want to light up, including ashtrays, matches, and vintage lighters. Clear out the oven. Do anything active and constructive. The moment you resist the urge AND have something to show for it, you'll feel better about yourself.

* Include fun in your daily schedule. The toughest thing you

will ever try to do may be to stop smoking. Celebrate your victories with enjoyable activities. You don't need to spend a lot of money, but you do need to take as much pleasure in the process as you can. Attend a movie. Visit the window stores. Visit some of the local tourist attractions. Visit a gallery or a museum. While you are preserving your life, keep yourself engaged!

* Involve others in your effort to stop smoking. Avoid being alone. Your decision will probably make your family and friends happy, and they'll want to support you. Spend some time mending damaged bonds. Invite a friend to a meal at a restaurant. Send the youngsters on an unique excursion. Take your significant other out on a date. Compared to when you were smoking, you can now travel places!

* Do not ever experience stress. Understand what makes you anxious, disturbed, or furious. Create a strategy for how you'll handle those circumstances without smoking if you can't totally avoid them. Practice deep breathing techniques. Take up meditation. Regular exercise Discover techniques to relieve tension and stress, and you'll soon be a successful non-smoker.

One strategy to stop smoking and regain that youthful glow is to include a regular workout regimen in your life. Exercise is an essential component of any attempt to stop smoking, while it definitely isn't a panacea.

Sports For Fun And Fitness

When you hear the phrase "sports fitness," what comes to mind? Do you witness tennis matches, volleyball teams at the beach, football players on the field, or soccer players squabbling over a ball? The phrase is frequently taken to refer to the sport itself rather than a method of exercise.

People play sports for a variety of recreational purposes, such as enjoyment, rivalry, or self-gratification. Most fitness gurus and medical professionals are aware that sports are one strategy to stay physically fit and healthy because they require physical exercise. But unlike "exercise" or "physical fitness," sports fitness entails honing a skill or aptitude. Fitness through sports offers a chance for personal development.

Because of the inherent discipline and physical demands of sports, sports aficionados may be more inclined to maintain a healthy lifestyle (although others would contest that claim). But in addition to losing weight and improving mobility and energy levels, sports fitness can also refer to a variety of other concepts we use to refer to good health. Sports fitness is a pursuit that develops moral character.

People are taught to respect their health through sports. They couldn't participate if they didn't have the energy and vitality to do so. Their fitness and health may be crucial to their livelihood, particularly if they play professional sports. Sporting fitness is a way of life.

Let's pretend for a moment that you are someone who requires more exercise to become or maintain physical health and fitness. Exercise at home, in gyms, or in health facilities are all options. You can exercise aerobically, follow a weight-training regimen, or spend hours on a treadmill or exercise bike. All of those are constructive pursuits. However, some of us find them dull. We won't follow them because we aren't enjoying them. Sport exercise is enjoyable!

The pursuit of sports fitness is one way to become healthy and have fun at the same time. On the baseball diamond or the basketball court, you can work out. You can compete in swimming events or marathons. These workouts include social connection, other people, and FUN! Let's assume that you have made the decision to acquire your exercise through sports fitness.

You should be aware of the following to ensure that sports fitness is a safe and healthy program for you:

1. Drink a lot of water

Without eating, we might go for days or even months. But we require regular access to drinking water to survive. It is the most significant nutrient we will ever eat. Additionally, you sweat more when you are exercising, losing that priceless liquid gold. In fact, if you lose too much fluid without replenishing it, it could seriously harm your health. At its worst, you might pass away.

Therefore, you should always drink water to replace what you lose via sweat when you engage in severe exercise. Some sports cause rapid fluid loss, making it unable to replenish them with just water. In reality, consuming excessive amounts of plain water at once might cause a hazardous reaction (water intoxication) because of an improper electrolyte balance in the body. Sports drinks are advised by specialists to prevent dehydration and water intoxication when participating in sports. They are divided into three groups.

Isotonic sports drinks have a comparable ratio of 6-8% sugar to water and other nutrients as the human body. Sports beverages that are hypertonic have higher sugar and lower water content than the human body. Sports drinks that are hypotonic have more water and less sugar than a human body. The majority of commercial sports beverages are isotonic.

Whatever you decide, sports drinks all contain electrolytes and carbs, which are vital components that aren't present in regular water. Energy levels are maintained by carbohydrates, and overall health depends on the right balance of electrolytes, which are composed of sodium, potassium, calcium, magnesium, chloride, phosphate, and hydrogen carbonate. Fluid intake is crucial for maintaining fitness for sports.

2. Increase your fruit and vegetable intake.

Sports-related physical exertion quickly depletes the body of vital vitamins and minerals. Important nutrients can be found in fruits and vegetables. Make it a habit to consume a dark green vegetable, a yellow or orange fruit or vegetable, a red fruit or vegetable, beans or nuts, and a citrus fruit like oranges every day when you're participating in a sports training program. A healthy, balanced diet is necessary for athletic fitness.

3. Guard your bones.

Those who are physically active in sports are obviously more likely to sustain injuries, such as shattered bones. The better off you will be, the more you can do to maintain strong bones. Make sure to eat foods high in calcium, such as dairy products, sardines, and tofu. Consider using a calcium supplement in your regular regimen as well. You'll not only be able to survive the knocks and bruises you receive on the court or field, but you'll also be giving your body a head start in fighting the terrible osteoporosis.

4. Preparation and Closing

If your body isn't flexible and limber when you start playing any kind of strenuous sport, you could strain a muscle or suffer another form of injury. Stretching exercises are a great way to get limber, just like running. Additionally, more vigorous warm-ups gradually increase your heart rate.

Don't head straight to the clubhouse or bar after the game. To gradually relieve tension and transition to less activity, perform a few cool-down exercises. If you do, your muscles are less tight and sore. Fitness for sports requires thoughtful planning and execution.

Sports participation is a terrific method to become and stay physically healthy as well as to lead an engaging, busy social life. You can meet more active individuals interested in health and fitness through sports, and they can help you stay motivated and involved. Sports fitness is the finest since it gives you a terrific exercise while having fun. The finest of both worlds is here!

Buyer Beware: Don't Buy These Elliptical Trainers

Be Wary of These Elliptical Trainers, Buyers

Finding reviews and suggestions for the top elliptical trainers is simple. You may learn about the devices that performed the best in their tests from a number of online consumer sites. But attempt to identify the equipment that is a waste of your money! You may attempt.

You might be shocked to find which manufacturers failed to deliver on elliptical trainers. There are certain elliptical trainers available created by reputable, well-known brands, but if you end up with one of them, you might as well flush your money down the toilet. We're here to let you know about the exercise equipment with poor elliptical trainer ratings so you can avoid wasting time, money, and heartache.

The Nordic Track brand is well-known. You wouldn't believe that a company so well recognized in the industry for their high-quality, affordably priced fitness equipment could also sell true garbage. You can, though. This is as a result of the CX925's shoddy construction, despite its numerous bells and whistles. This machine boasts a lot of highly appealing features, including a stylish LED dashboard panel, the flexibility to adjust the slope, and the opportunity to choose from a variety of programs. Even though many customers were generally happy with their equipment, they also mentioned numerous mechanical issues and pricey repairs. This model was rated below average for both durability and display by EllipticalTrainers.com. The main line is that even though you may get a lot of upscale features for a reasonable price, you definitely shouldn't count on them lasting very long. You'll waste a lot of time waiting while also having to spend a lot of money on repairs. The Nordic Track AudioStrider 990, on the other hand, received a Best Buy rating from Consumer Reports in its category.

Another well-known company with a solid reputation is ProForm. However, their 900 elliptical received poor reviews and had several severe issues. What we discovered is that ProForm machines that aren't part of their EFX line just aren't as good as we had thought. The 90-day warranties are too short and point to a limited product life, despite the affordable price and little noise. Some customers complained about the manufacturer's poor customer service and support as well as numerous small breaks that render the equipment useless. They added that not all the parts were included in the package and that it was challenging to build. By creating a more straightforward version of their EFX models, ProForm has proven that they are capable of creating a superior machine. But they made the decision not to. The ProForm XP 520 Razor is a wonderful option if you're seeking for a low cost. Despite receiving the worst ratings out of eight elliptical trainer reviews,

According to ConsumerReports.org, it was far less expensive than every other device they examined. Therefore, we suggest that you search elsewhere if you are not investing in a ProForm EFX model.

Some of the lowest scores for elliptical trainers were given to Horizon. These Chinese-made machines aren't made for everyone because they have some of the shortest strides in the business. The machines were unpleasant and unreliable. Horizon, sadly, doesn't seem to provide a high-quality product since they rely on employing inexpensive materials. They seem to be attempting to outbid rival Vision for cheap costs. However, EllipticalTrainers.com cautions that regular cleaning is necessary to keep their equipment in working order since it soon becomes dusty.

Despite their low cost, you can spend the same amount of money on a superior machine. We have found very little favorable information on the Horizon elliptical trainers, thus we strongly advise that you go for another brand instead.

So what can we learn from this? If you're considering purchasing exercise equipment, check for the elliptical trainers with the highest ratings that have been reviewed by reliable, well-known experts.

With that fantastic offer, you could believe you're saving a ton of money, but you're more likely to get a machine that doesn't perform what you need it to do, breaks the moment you use it, and ends up costing you more in consumer angst than it ever did in savings.

To be clear, we're not knocking Nordic Track or ProForm for producing quality goods. It's true. Simply do your research and make sure you're purchasing the suggested models. When choosing from glowing customer reviews and excellent ratings, you can rely on elliptical trainer ratings to help you make the greatest purchases. Make sure to check out what customers have to say about their devices as well. It belongs to you. You can decide. Now get out and start exercising!

Water And Exercise

The greatest quote is from poet W.H. Auden: "Thousands have lived without love, but not one without water."

The human body contains up to 75% water. Without water, people can't survive. In actuality, we are only able to survive without water for three days. Water is the most essential nutrient in our life when you take into account how long we can go without it. It's critical to keep in mind that water is not only beneficial to health, but also essential for living a longer, higher-quality life.

The amount of water any person needs depends largely on their lifestyle, weight, and climate. Those who work out frequently require extra water. Those who are heavier require more water. In arid climates, people require extra water. According to research, more than two-thirds of Americans don't get the recommended amount of water each day. Your body is replenished and kept hydrated when you drink enough water, which enables it to perform as it should.

Our blood transports nutrients and oxygen throughout our bodies, and water eliminates waste when we urinate or sweat. Water is crucial for healthy joints. Water also enables us to digest food even if it has no energy value.

Most people only consume water when they are thirsty. The

greatest way to determine your body's demands is not to wait until you become thirsty. Actually, we don't feel thirsty until after we've been dehydrated. Fatigue is frequently caused by dehydration. Additionally, it can cause a number of minor symptoms like headaches, lightheadedness, low blood pressure, and others. Dehydration can, at its worst, cause hallucinations, unconsciousness, or even death.

People should generally consume at least 2 liters (or 8 cups) of water per day. People who exercise, are heavier, or reside in arid climates should consume enough liquid to make up for the water they lose via sweat. You might assume that any beverage would suffice to satisfy your water requirements. However, that is untrue. Other beverages, such as sodas, coffee, and alcohol, which function as diuretics and make us urinate more when we consume them, may even cause your body to lose water. In reality, even though you may believe that drinking these kinds of beverages gives you more water, you actually lose it almost as quickly as you take it in.

More water is required. when you work out. You sweat when you work out or work out, which speeds up the rate at which your body loses water. This holds true in both cold and warm climates. Professionals urge us to consume 1-2 cups of water before working out and to keep doing so during the entire exercise. You should consume at least 16 ounces (two cups) of water for each pound of weight you lose through exercise.

Even when you sleep, water is lost from your body. A glass or two of water before bed will make you more awake and alert in the morning. A major justification for consuming more water than normal is illness. Our bodies quickly lose water when we have the flu or a cold, which makes us feel much worse. By consuming more water while you're sick, you can aid in preventing this.

Whether bottled water is superior to tap water is a topic of popular discussion. In fact, the government has strict regulations in place for tap water. Your local water system's tap water is safe to drink unless it isn't in conformity with laws. On the other side, there are fewer restrictions on bottled water. Of course, bottled water is significantly more expensive than tap water. However, you should conduct your own research to determine which type of water best suits your needs.

Drink a glass or two of water several times per day to live a long, healthy life. Drink water throughout the day and carry water with you whenever you can. Developing the habit of drinking water instead of other beverages that don't replace your body's nutrition is also a smart suggestion.

Water is essential for both life and wellness. One simple method to ensure a long, healthy life is to establish and maintain good behaviors. Remember to consume two liters or more of water each day. Drink more than two liters if you are active.

How Can I Find The Best Elliptical Trainer?

If you're looking for a new elliptical trainer, you probably already know that there are a bewildering variety of brands and designs available. How do you decide what to do?

You're off base if you think it's only an issue of preference or opinion. In truth, the best elliptical trainers are routinely provided by a highly regarded brand.

The items produced by Precor demonstrate their commitment to becoming the most reputable company in exercise equipment. According to ellipticaltrainers.com, Precor invented the elliptical cross trainer first and has since "established the standard for quality, high-end elliptical trainers." The EFX was the name of the original elliptical machine, and it is still in use today.

Although the EFX series from Precor has a range of features and costs, they all share ease of use. Your workout will be more pleasurable and efficient if the equipment is simple to use because you won't have to spend time figuring it out.

The EFX is even lower impact than other machines on the market, despite the fact that most elliptical trainers are low-impact, moderate exercise equipment. Even if you are reaping the rewards of a challenging workout without being exhausted, your workout feels easy. The Precor EFX series' simplicity of use makes it ideal for beginners and almost mislead you into thinking you're not working. You can change the muscle groups you're working on and adjust the incline thanks to their patented CrossRamp feature. Additionally, because their trainers have no weight restriction, they are suitable for heavier users.

A remarkable 10-year warranty, rarely provided by other manufacturers in the sector, is included with Precor's EFX. Consumers concur that Precor's warranty demonstrates their confidence in the dependability and quality of their elliptical trainers. They have discovered that the EFX series has a long product life and requires almost no maintenance. They do not offer a cheap EFX series. They may be the most expensive on the market, costing between $3000 and $5000. However, consumerreports.org gave them the top spot and gave them 100 percent on the four comparison criteria of ergonomics, construction, exercise range, and ease of use. Elliptical trainers made by Precor are top-of-the-line items that fulfill all of their promises.

Elliptical trainers from Precor move the way you do. With the aid of ergonomic handlebars, you can keep both good form and comfort while conditioning your entire body. With 20 resistance levels and synchronized handlebars, a variety of programs are available for more varied workouts and quicker results. No matter your level of fitness, you can get a fun workout that gives you the outcomes you want.

For more than 20 years, Precor has offered high-quality training equipment. They are a developing, environmentally responsible, and ethical manufacturer with arguably the best reputation for quality and value in the sector. You owe it to yourself to look into Precor's EFX series if you're looking to get an elliptical trainer

www.ingramcontent.com/pod-product-compliance
Lightning Source LLC
Chambersburg PA
CBHW071213260726
48653CB00041B/252